Breast Sonography
A Comprehensive Sonographer's Guide

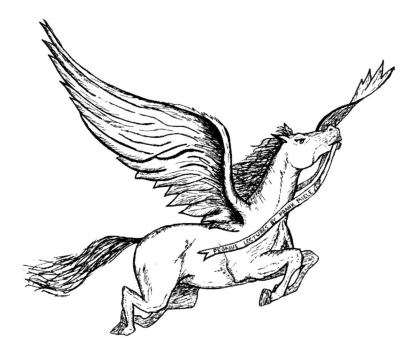

Pegasus Lectures, Inc.

Catherine Carr-Hoefer
RT, RDMS, RDCS, RVT, FSDMS

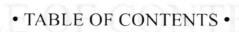

• TABLE OF CONTENTS •

• CHAPTER ONE •

Breast Sonography Instrumentation

A. Transducer Selection and Features

Features of a transducer suitable for high-resolution breast imaging include:
- Linear array format
- High frequency
- Broad bandwidth
- Variable electronic focusing
- Near-field focusing
- Thin slice thickness

Ultrasound systems used for breast imaging require excellent:
- Spatial resolution
- Contrast resolution

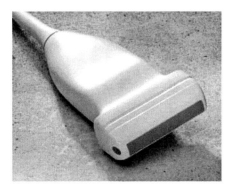

1. Linear Array Format

A linear array transducer has a rectangular shape and image field. Side-by-side piezoelectric crystals are activated in groups that are then sequenced to produce parallel scan lines that provide a uniform image field from near to far fields. Phased array linear transducers use both sequencing and electronic phasing to create, focus, and steer the sound beam.

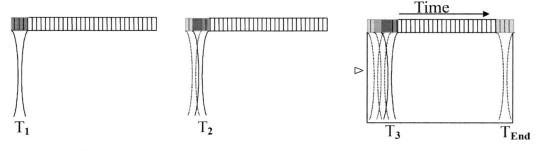

(Schematic reprinted with permission from SDMS/Pegasus Breast Ultrasound Exam Simulation CD, 2003)

Benefits of linear array format
- Rectangular shape allows direct skin contact and even compression of the underlying tissues.
- Sound beam incidence is more perpendicular to the skin and chest wall for more uniform imaging during breast examination.
- Wide acoustic window in the near-field allows better demonstration of superficial structures without beam divergence.
- Uniform image field and less beam divergence allows more accurate measurement of breast masses.
- Narrow focusing characteristics improve needle visualization during interventional procedures.

2. High-Frequency

High frequency is needed for optimal breast imaging because of the superficial location of the breast and the need to resolve small structures.

> Center frequency 10 MHz or higher   (ACR Practice Guidelines 10/07)*
> *ACR = American College of Radiology*

Most high-resolution real-time transducers span a range of frequencies that can exceed 10 MHz.

Key advantage of using high frequency:
- Improved axial resolution
  (Axial resolution = ability to differentiate two closely spaced echo interfaces lying in the direction of the sound beam.)

Disadvantage of using high frequency:
- Reduced penetration secondary to more rapid attenuation of the sound beam

Technical Note: Choose a frequency high enough to obtain maximum detail of breast structures while still allowing adequate sound penetration of the region of interest.

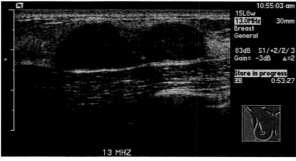

13.0 MHz.
Poor sound penetration of mass and chest wall.

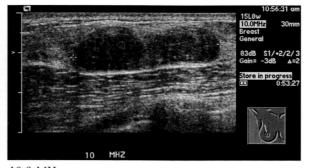

10.0 MHz.
Better sound penetration of mass and chest wall.

3. Broad Bandwidth

A pulsed-wave transducer produces a sound beam that contains more than one frequency. Besides the center operating (resonant) frequency, a spectrum of other higher and lower frequencies is generated, called the bandwidth.

Bandwidth and pulse length are inversely proportional. High-resolution transducers used for breast imaging emit short pulses of sound that generate a wide range of frequencies. Broader bandwidths improves spatial and contrast resolution, and enhance image quality. To shorten the pulse length, a damping material is placed behind the transducer to reduce ringing of the transducer elements.

2

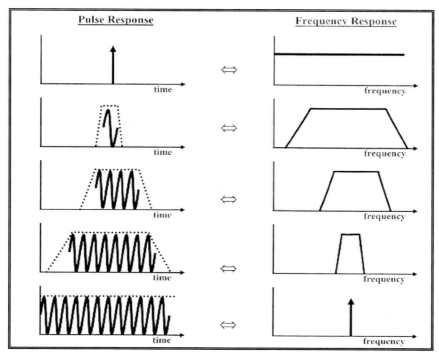

Pulse Response	Frequency Response
time	frequency

Pulse Length   *Bandwidth*

When broadband systems are used, an operating frequency of 10 MHz or higher is optimum.

Advantages of broad bandwidth transducers:
- Transducer can operate at different frequencies to optimize resolution or sound penetration (multi-hertz control)
- Allows B-mode transmission at higher frequency, while simultaneously performing spectral and color Doppler at lower frequency
- Allows harmonic imaging with transmission of the sound beam at a lower fundamental frequency and reception of the sound beam at a higher harmonic frequency

4. **Beam Focusing**

The ultrasound beam of a transducer is 3-dimensional. Focusing affects the width and thickness of the sound beam. A narrower sound beam improves resolution and intensifies sound energy at the focus.

Lateral resolution is best where the sound beam is narrowest, which is at the focus.
(Lateral resolution = the ability to resolve two closely spaced interfaces lying side-by-side in a direction perpendicular to the sound beam.)

Beam focusing features of a conventional 1-D linear phased-array transducer include:

Variable Electronic Focusing
- Focusing that occurs along the long axis of a linear array transducer (in the lateral plane)
- Focusing can be altered at various distances from the transducer by altering/delaying the timing of excitation of the transducer elements
- Multiple transmit foci create a narrower transmit beam
- Continuous receive focus creates a narrow receive beam
- Improves lateral resolution

Fixed Elevation Focus   (1-D linear arrays)
- Represents focusing along the short axis of the transducer
- Fixed focal depth at ~1.5cm for high frequency breast transducer
- Achieved by use of acoustic lens
- Corresponds to slice thickness perpendicular to the scan plane
- Elevational resolution is best at the elevation focal depth
  (Elevational resolution is determined by the beamwidth in the elevation plane.)

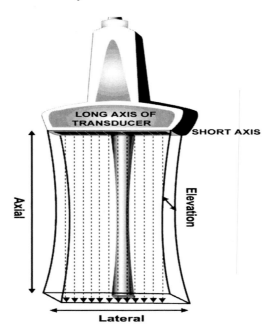

Modified from Miele F. Ultrasound Physics & Instrumentation. 4th Ed. Miele Enterprises, LLC, 2006.

A shallow elevation focus (elevation plane) of a high frequency, linear array transducer improves near field detail and reduces slice thickness. For a conventional 1-dimensional, linear-array transducer, the short-axis plane of focus is fixed at a depth selected by the manufacturer based on the utility of the transducer. For example, a 6 MHz linear array transducer designed for vascular imaging will have a deeper elevation plane focus than a 10 MHz linear array transducer designed for breast imaging.
(1.5-D and matrix array transducers are available on some newer systems that allow variable electronic focusing in both elevation and lateral planes.)

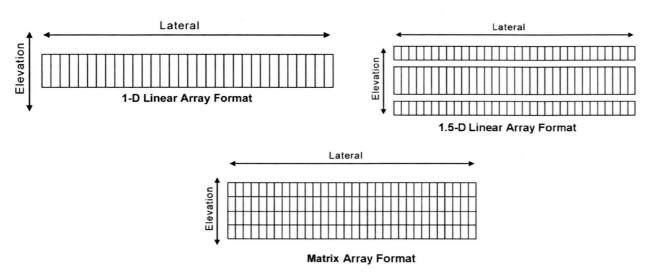

Adapted from Miele F. Ultrasound Physics & Instrumentation. 4th Ed. Miele Enterprises, LLC

B. Resolution

High-frequency, broad bandwidth transducers provide excellent spatial and contrast resolution. Resolution refers to the size of the smallest object depicted on the ultrasound image given adequate contrast.

Spatial and contrast resolution impacts image quality and the ability to detect small and subtle breast structures and pathology.

1. Spatial (Detail) Resolution

Spatial resolution refers to the US system's ability to accurately depict very small anatomic structures at their correct location on the image.

Spatial resolution for an ultrasound system is measured in 3 planes:
- Axial plane   (along the direction of sound beam)
- Lateral plane   (perpendicular to the sound beam)
- Elevation plane   (perpendicular to the sound beam; corresponds to the slice thickness)

Generally, spatial resolution is best in the axial plane where resolution is better than 1mm. Spatial resolution is primarily affected by transducer characteristics (frequency, focusing, scan lines), as well system electronics and the display resolution.

Axial resolution improves with:
- Higher frequency transducers
- Shorter pulse lengths
- Broader bandwidth transducers

2. Contrast Resolution

Contrast resolution is the ability of the ultrasound system to distinguish anatomic structures based on variations in echo brightness. This refers to both the ability of the system to differentiate tissues with slightly different echo amplitudes (low contrast resolution), as well as large differences in echo amplitudes (high contrast resolution). Contrast resolution is improved when the ultrasound system can recognize and store in memory a wide range of differences in echo strength. Excellent contrast resolution is especially important when trying to detect a subtle, isoechoic lesion in the fatty breast.

Some factors affecting contrast resolution include:
- Scan converter (#bits/pixel)   (Digital scan converters greatly extend dynamic range.)
- Acoustic impedance mismatch
- Transducer frequency
- Post processing curves
- Dynamic range
- Signal-to-noise ratio
- Artifacts
- Monitor brightness and contrast settings

Contrast resolution impacts spatial resolution. If a system has poor contrast resolution, two closely spaced objects may appear as one.

3. Temporal Resolution

Temporal resolution is the ability of the ultrasound system to distinguish moving objects, or dynamics over time. In most situations, temporal resolution is not severely affected during breast imaging because of the limited depth of field needed to study superficial organs.

Temporal resolution is limited by the FRAME RATE. Factors that affect frame rate include:
- Imaging depth (scale)
- Number of focal zones
- Image size
- Line density
- Number of acoustic lines per display line (packet size in color)
- Use of parallel processing
- Compound imaging
- Combined 2D/Doppler (Duplex; Triplex Imaging)

C. System Controls and Optimization

Equipment parameters that need to be optimized during the breast sonographic examination include:
- Output power
- Overall gain
- Time Gain Compensation
- Dynamic range
- Focal zone placement and number
- Frame rate
- Image scale
- Monitor brightness and contrast
- Other knobology

Brightness of the echoes on the ultrasound image are affected by:
- Output power
- Overall gain
- Time Gain Compensation
- Dynamic Range
- (Monitor Settings)

1. Output Power

Output power affects the amplitude of the transmit voltage, and therefore, the intensity of the transmitted sound beam.

Terms used:

• Output power	• Transmit power
• Acoustic power	• Transmit gain
• Power gain	• Transmit voltage
• Power setting	• Output voltage
• Acoustic gain	• Output intensity

The output power controls the excitation voltage that drives the transducer crystals. A higher voltage corresponds to a higher mechanical oscillation of the crystal elements, and subsequently, a higher amplitude sound wave that generates brighter echoes.

↑ output power →
   ↑ voltage to transducer crystals →
      ↑ mechanical oscillation of crystals →
         ↑ amplitude (intensity) of transmitted sound beam →
            ↑ ultrasound energy received by patient

Pegasus Lectures, Inc.

When the output power is increased, a higher intensity sound beam is transmitted and reflected back to the receiver. A higher intensity beam produces a larger signal (greater signal to noise ratio) and improves the system's ability to detect signals from weak reflectors and deep structures.

Technical notes:

The power setting should be adjusted so that all breast tissues are adequately penetrated from the skin surface to the chest wall. Since the output power affects the intensity of the signal going to the patient, excessive settings should be avoided (ALARA principle).

2. **Overall Gain (Receiver Gain)**

    The overall gain control provides uniform amplification of all of the echo signals returning to the transducer. This is a receiver gain control and does NOT affect the intensity of the sound beam transmitted by the transducer.

    Since the returning echo signals are weak (due to attenuation) as compared to the transmitted signals, the returning signals must be electronically amplified for proper image processing.

    Increasing receiver gain increases the overall brightness (amplitude) of the echoes of the ultrasound image. Decreasing receiver gain decreases the overall brightness of the echoes.

    Technical notes:

    Gain settings are operator dependent. For breast imaging, the overall gain should be adjusted to ensure adequate demonstration of all true echoes. For breast imaging, gain settings and dynamic range should be set so breast fat displays a medium-level gray shade. Excessive gain settings will introduce false echoes within breast tissues and cysts. Too low of a gain setting will reduce detection of real echoes and can make a solid mass appear cystic.

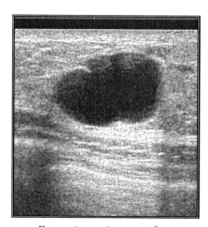 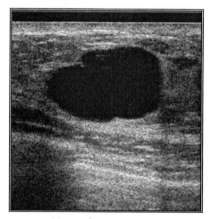 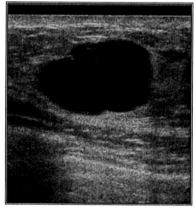

Excessive gain = artifacts   *Normal gain setting*   *Low gain = miss echoes*

3. **Time Gain Compensation**

    The time gain compensation (TGC) control allows selective amplification of weaker echo signals from deep structures to compensate for attenuation losses. The TGC is an operator dependent, receiver gain control.

    Correct adjustment of the TGC will make a nonuniform image appear more uniform. The degree of echo amplification can be altered at different depths by sliding individual TGC pods or adjusting near-to-far field control knobs.

Technical note:
The TGC should be adjusted so all echoes reflected from similar structures are displayed with the same brightness (amplitude) from near-to-far fields. For example, the subcutaneous fat should display the same grayshade level as the retromammary fat.

Modern ultrasound systems "pre-adjust" the TCG for a specific exam preset, so the TCG setting may appear linear.

4. **Dynamic Range**
The displayed dynamic range of an ultrasound system is the range from the lowest grayscale level to the maximum grayscale brightness level on the image. Dynamic range affects contrast resolution. Displayed dynamic range and grayscale processing allows echoes of varying amplitudes to be displayed on the image.

Technically, dynamic range is defined as the ratio of the smallest to the largest signal strength level that the system can handle without distortion. The number of gray shades that an ultrasound system displays is adjusted by the dynamic range, compression, or reject controls.

Technical note:
Increasing the dynamic range will allow a greater range of echoes to be displayed (increasing grayscale levels). This allows demonstration of more subtle differences in tissue echogenicity. Decreasing dynamic range will make the ultrasound image appear more contrasty and will show less differentiation of gray scale patterns.

5. **Focal Zone Placement and Number**
The "focus" control allows the sonographer to adjust the placement and the number of transmit focal zones within the breast.

As mentioned earlier, electronic focusing narrows the beamwidth along the long axis of the transducer and improves lateral resolution. (The fixed short-axis elevation plane focus cannot be manually adjusted when using a conventional linear array transducer.)

Technical notes:
The number and depth of the focal zones must be set appropriately during breast imaging. For general breast imaging, a single transmit focus should be placed in the mid-to-deep breast. The depth of focus is usually ≤ 3cm. When examining a breast mass, the focal zone should be set at a depth corresponding to the midportion of the mass. Improper focusing can cause false echoes from volume averaging.

Using multiple transmit foci allows a narrow transmit beam over a greater depth in the breast. In general, three or less focal zones provide adequate focusing throughout the depth of the breast.

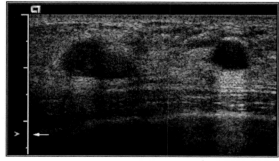

Focus set too deep resulting in poor mass delineation and false echoes within the cyst.

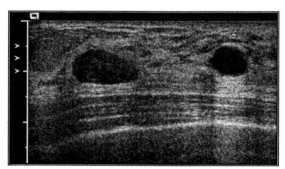

Multiple focal zones at level of mass improve lesion clarity and reduces detrimental artifacts.

Pegasus Lectures, Inc.

6. **Frame Rate**

Frame rate is the number of images displayed per second and affects temporal resolution. The sonographer alters the frame rate when changing the number of focal zones, the image depth and the frame size or by adding functions such as compounding imaging or Doppler.

Technical note:

During breast imaging, using multiple transmit foci significantly slows frame rate. To help compensate for this, reducing image depth or image size to the area of interest can improve frame rates.

7. **Image Scale**

The size and depth of the image shown on the display monitor can be altered during breast imaging by the sonographer. Increasing image depth allows deeper structures to be viewed. Decreasing image depth optimizes visualization of superficial structures. Maximum image depth depends on the specific transducer.

Technical notes:

For general imaging, the image depth should be set so all layers of the breast are seen from the skin to the chest wall. If the image depth is set too deep, the image will appear too small on the display.

Enlarging the field-of-view (magnification, "write zoom", RES-mode) is important when evaluating the margin characteristics and the internal features of a breast mass.

8. **Other Knobology**

Other system controls that need to be optimized during breast imaging include:
- Pre- and post processing
- Persistence (affects frame averaging)
- Doppler settings
- Monitor brightness and contrast

New systems provide "image optimization" buttons that automatically set and update controls such as the gain, TGC, and focus based on exam preset, image depth, and tissue type.

D. **Doppler**

Doppler allows the noninvasive detection of blood flow within vessels, masses and tissues. Doppler modes used in breast imaging include:

1. **Pulsed-waved Spectral Doppler**
- Blood flow sampling at a selected depth within a vessel segment
- Spectral waveform displays changes in the flow velocity and direction of moving red blood cells over a period of time
- Blood flow detection is angle dependent
- Waveform pattern differentiates arterial from venous flow
- Waveform pattern differentiates turbulent from laminar flow
- Measurements include peak, mean, and minimal flow velocities, and RI, PI values
- High velocities are subject to aliasing
- Audio component correlates with spectral tracing

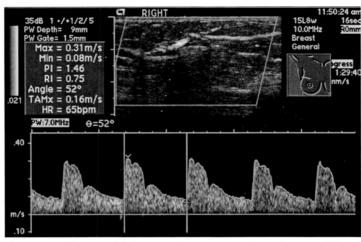

Triplex image showing 2D grayscale, power-mode and spectral Doppler.
Spectral waveform confirms that the tubular breast structure is an artery.

2. **Color flow Doppler**
   - Superimposed color display of blood flow on anatomic grayscale image
   - Multiple sample gates along each scan line determine average flow rate (mean velocity) and flow direction
   - Rapid identification of blood flow in vessels / masses
   - Detection of blood vessels too small to be seen on B-mode image
   - Demonstration of complex flow patterns (turbulence)
   - Flow detection is angle dependent
     (Detection is optimized when blood flow is parallel to the sound beam. No flow is detected when blood flow direction is perpendicular to the sound beam.)
   - High velocities can cause mosaic of colors from aliasing

3. **Power (angio) Doppler**
   - Estimates the total strength (amplitude, intensity) of the Doppler shift within each gated region. (Relies on the number, not the velocity, of the moving red blood cells.)
   - Less angle dependent
   - Better sensitivity to low flow states
   - Better demonstration of tortuous and small vessels
   - No information on flow direction, velocity, or turbulence
   - No aliasing, but more susceptible to motion artifacts

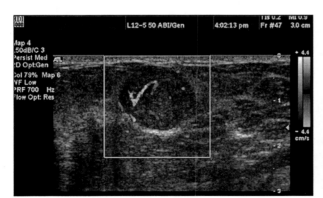

Color Doppler Image of solid breast mass.
(Courtesy: Philips Medical Systems)

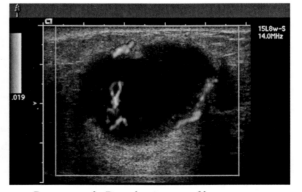

Power-mode Doppler image of breast mass
(Courtesy: Siemens Medical)

Technical Notes:

Doppler settings should be optimized for low flow states:

- Decrease PRF setting enough to detect flow without aliasing
- Optimize velocity scale
- Use low flow filter
- Use enough gain to detect flow signal without introducing artifact
- Optimize Doppler angle (for spectral and Color-flow)
- Use minimal transducer pressure (so as not to compress vessels)

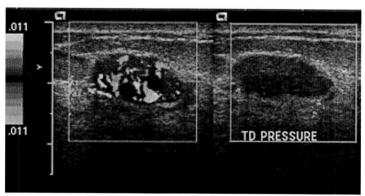

Light transducer pressure helps to optimize blood flow detection.
Heavy transducer pressure reduces blood flow detection.

4. Doppler - Contrast Agents

In the United States, the Food and Drug Administration (FDA) does not currently approve intravenous contrast agents for breast ultrasound applications. However, some American research centers and facilities outside the USA are using stabilized microbubble contrast agents to evaluate tumor vascularity.

The ultrasound pulse causes the microbubbles to vibrate causing the emission of harmonic frequencies. The ultrasound system listens for the harmonic signals generated from the US contrast agent.

The presence of microbubbles in blood increases the acoustic backscatter, which increases the amplitude of the returning sound waves. The enhanced Doppler signal allows detection of weaker echoes received from blood flowing in small blood vessels. This allows better assessment of tumor neovascularity.

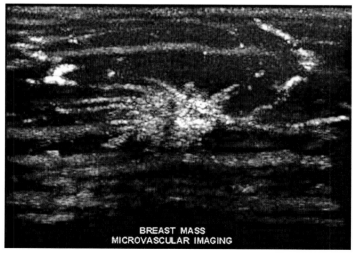

Microbubble contrast agent provides enhanced detection of blood flow within this breast mass.
(Courtesy: Philips Medical Systems)

E. Specialty Applications

1. Split-Screen Imaging

This application allows two ultrasound images to be placed side-by-side on the image display. This dual-mode format is helpful for showing the size of larger masses. Side-by-side imaging allows comparison of breast segments and implants at similar levels in each breast; demonstration of a lesion's appearance and measurements in orthogonal scan planes, as well as, dynamic compression effects.

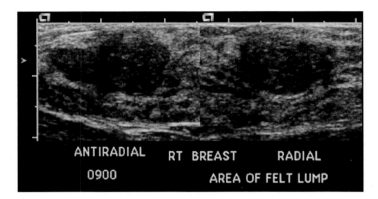

2. Extended-Field-of-View (EFOV)

This technique allows a real-time ultrasound scan to be acquired and displayed over a longer distance across the breast than that achievable with conventional imaging. EFOV allows better documentation of the size and spatial extent of pathologic lesions and of normal anatomic structures.

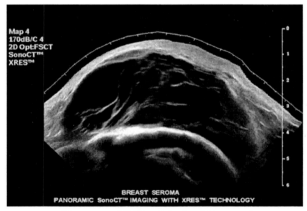

(Courtesy: Philips Medical Systems)

3. Tissue Harmonic Imaging

As sound travels through the body, the ultrasound wave becomes distorted as it propagates through tissues with varying densities and other acoustic properties. As a result, the insonated tissues reflect sound back to the transducer at multiples of the transmitted frequency. Newer generation ultrasound systems with broadband technology can detect and process these subtle, higher frequency, harmonic signals.

During harmonic imaging, the ultrasound system transmits at a given (fundamental) frequency and selectively receives and processes harmonic echo signals that resonate from the tissues at twice the transmit (second harmonic) frequency.

Some advantages of tissue harmonic imaging include maintaining sound penetration when transmitting at the lower (fundamental) frequency, while achieving better resolution when receiving at the higher (harmonic) frequency. Lateral resolution improves since the harmonic beam is narrower than the fundametal sound beam. Additionally, harmonic imaging significantly reduces artifacts (reverberation, speckle, clutter) and improves contrast resolution. These artifacts are typically related to transmission at the fundamental frequency and are often generated close to the skin or body wall. Harmonic imaging reduces or eliminates many of the false echoes seen in breast cysts and masses, and enhances margin delineation.

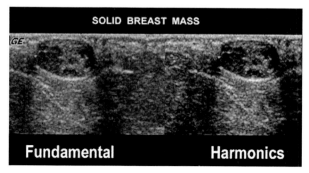

4. Spatial Compound Imaging

Real-time spatial compound imaging is a newer technique that provides a single compound image created from multiple scan planes transmitted sequentially from different angles. These angled scan planes produce an image that better defines margins of masses, subareolar structures, and reduces artifacts (reverberation, edge shadowing, speckle, noise).

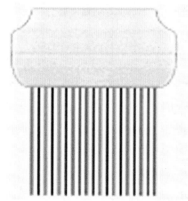 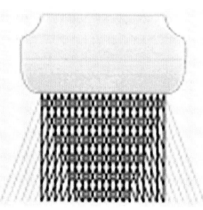

Conventional linear-array transducer.   *Compound image acquisition*
(Courtesy: Philips Medical Systems)

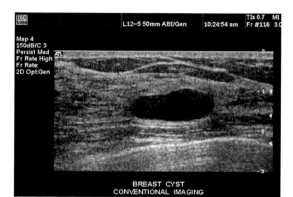 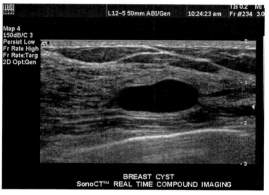

Conventional image with artifacts within cyst.   *Compound image with artifact reduction and better margin delineation.*

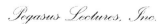

A pitfall to spatial compounding is the potential reduction of useful clinical markers such as distal shadowing and sound enhancement.

5. **Convex Linear (Trapezoidal) Imaging**
   Some linear transducers can electronically change the image shape from a rectangle to a "trapezoid" by pushing a control button, thus allowing a wider field-of-view.

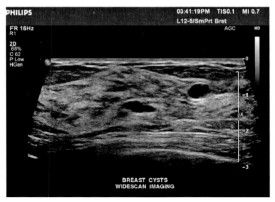

Image Courtesy: Philips Medical

6. **3D/4D Imaging; Multiplanar / Multi-slice Imaging**
   New-generation ultrasound scanners provide options for viewing breast tissues in 3 dimensions (X, Y, Z planes) allowing surface and volume rendering of masses. "Real-time" 3-D is referred to as 4-D imaging. Once a volume data set is acquired, a breast mass can be imaged in multidimensional planes or in a "slice-by-slice" format. Depending on the system, the volumetric data may be reviewed on a separate workstation allowing offline manipulation of the image data. (Some whole-breast automated breast scanners also provide these features.)

   The ability to view the coronal plane of a mass from a volume set obtained from standard views can enhance demonstration of malignant features such as spiculation.

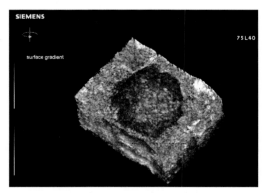

3D Surface Rendering: Solid microlobulated mass.
Images Courtesy: Siemen's Medical

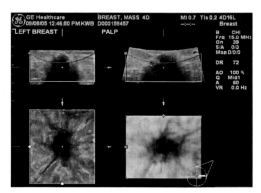

3D/4D Multi-plane image
of malignant mass with spiculation.
Image Courtesy: GE Healthcare

7. **Elasticity Imaging (Informational – Not likely to be on ARDMS exam)**
   Elasticity imaging is available on some new ultrasound systems. This technique uses differences in tissue deformation (strain) to create images of relative tissue stiffness during real-time imaging. Soft breast masses are compressible (elastic), whereas, hard masses are poorly compressible or "stiff." Soft lesions (e.g, fluid masses) tend to appear internally "white" on the elastogram image, whereas stiffer masses appear "black." Solid masses are relatively "stiff" compared to cystic lesions. On an elastogram, benign solid lesions tend to be smaller, whereas cancers tend to be larger than the size shown on a standard 2D B-mode image.

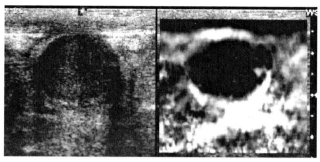
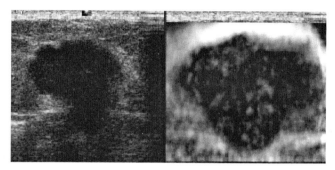

Benign fibdroadenoma. Elastogram (right) displays the mass as dark (stiff) with the lesion size being slightly smaller than on the conventional image.

Invasive ducatal carcinoma. Elastogram displays the cancer as dark (stiff) with the lesion size larger than on the conventional image.

Images Courtesy of Siemen's Medical

F. Artifacts

An artifact is any false information on the ultrasound image. An artifact does not correspond to a true anatomical structure. Understanding and recognizing artifacts is important to avoid misdiagnosis.

Artifacts can be caused by:
- Atypical sound interaction within the body
- Equipment deficiencies or malfunction
- Interfering signals
- Image processing
- Operator error
- Patient movement

1. Reverberation

- Represents multiple, repetitive reflections between two strong, specular reflectors. The reflectors are usually superficial in the breast.
- Due to the large acoustic mismatch, a large percentage of the beam is reflected, and then partially reflected back by the transducer.
- Artifact occurs when the sound beam is perpendicular to the interface.
- The "bouncing back and forth" between the transducer and the reflector increases travel time, causing the reverberating echoes to be displayed at different depths on the image.
- The reverberating echoes are seen as equally spaced lines of diminishing amplitude with depth.
- Reverberation is a common cause of false echoes within the anterior portion of cystic structures.

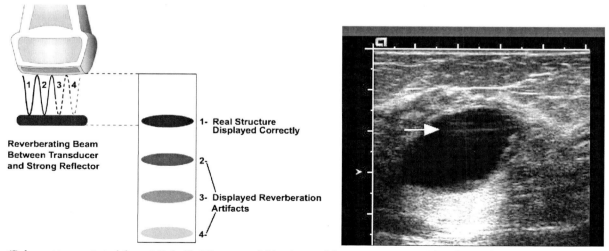

(Schematic reprinted from Miele F: Ultrasound Physics and Instrumentation, 4th Ed., Miele Enterprises, 2006.)

a. Comet-tail artifact
  - Type of reverberation; appears as multiple small parallel echo bands.
  - Usually caused by two closely spaced strong reflectors in soft-tissue.
  - Can be seen with surgical slips, biopsy needles.

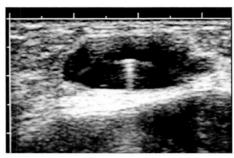

Cross-section of hollow needle within cyst causing comet-tail artifact.

b. Ring-down artifact
  - Type of reverberation; generally produced by small gas bubbles.
  - Seen at aperture opening of a vacuum-assisted breast biopsy device.

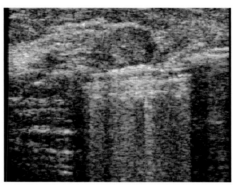

Ring-down artifact from Mammotome aperture.
(Courtesy: Cindy Rapp, BS, RDMS)

2. Enhancement
  - Form of attenuation artifact
  - Represents an increase in echo amplitude from interfaces that lie beneath a weakly-attenuating or non-attenuating structure.
  - Occurs beneath structures that are weak reflectors, or that absorb less sound than adjacent tissues at the same depth.
  - Since sound easily propagates through homogeneous, fluid-filled structures, such as breast cysts, there is more sound energy left to insonify distal structures. Distal echoes appear bright or "enhanced."

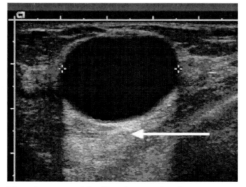

Simple cyst with distal sound enhancement.

3. Shadowing

- Attenuation artifact
- Represents a decrease in sound energy beneath a structure that attenuates more sound than adjacent tissues at the same depth.
- Both strong reflectors and strong absorbers will cause a decrease in sound beam intensity. This results in a region of "echo drop-out" beneath the attenuating structure.
- The greater the attenuation, the greater is the shadowing.

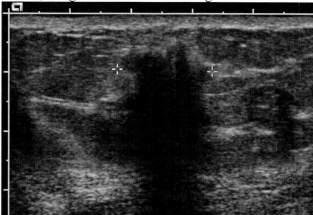

Shadowing breast mass.

4. Refraction

- Represents a change in the direction of the sound beam as it passes from one medium to another.
- Reflection appears improperly positioned laterally on the image.
- Occurs when there is a significant difference in propagation speeds at an acoustic interface, and when the sound beam is not perpendicular to the interface.

Refractive Edge Shadowing; Critical-angle Shadowing

- Bending of sound beam and loss of sound energy causing a shadow.
- Caused by refraction of the sound beam. Once the sound beam reaches a critical angle, little or no ultrasound energy transmits across the interface, creating a shadow.
- Encountered at curved edges of breast cysts and some solid masses, and with oblique incidence to Cooper's ligaments.

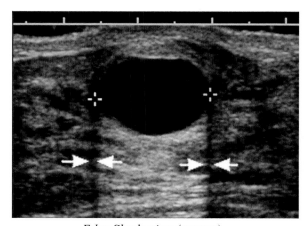

Edge Shadowing (arrows).

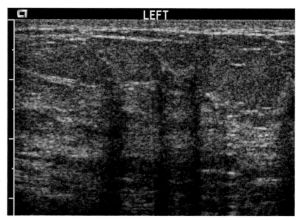

Critical angle shadowing from Cooper's ligaments.

5. Propagation Speed Error

- Represents incorrect registration of the depth of a structure on the image when the sound velocity through the structure is significantly different than the assumed velocity of 1540m/s for soft tissue.
- If the speed of sound is slower than in soft tissue, posterior echoes are registered on the ultrasound image deeper than in reality. For example, this artifact occurs when sound travels though silicone (speed of sound ~ 1000m/s).
- If the speed of sound is significantly faster than in soft tissue, reflectors will be placed closer to the transducer than in reality.

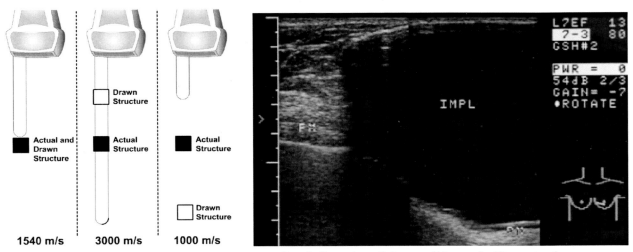

Depth distortion of chest wall beneath silicone implant.
(Schematic reprinted from Miele F: Ultrasound Physics and Instrumentation, 4th Ed., Miele Enterprises, 2006.)

Bayonet sign = "broken-needle" artifact can be seen during needle-guidance related to the difference in the speed of sound between the needle and the surrounding tissue interface. This artifact confirms that the needle is within the cyst/mass.

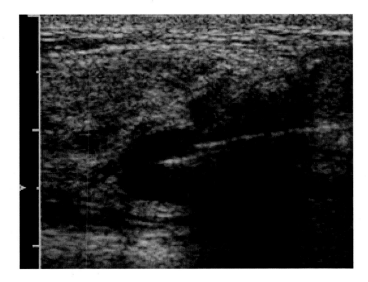

6. Side Lobes; Grating Lobes

- Side lobes are weaker sound beams from a single element transducer directed in regions other than the main beam axis.
- Grating lobes are extra beams emitted from a multi-element transducer array. Grating lobes are the result of partial constructive (or destructive) interference.
- Reflections from acoustic energy directed in regions other than the main beam axis adds with the energy of the main beam reflection causing spurious echoes that degrade the image.
- Side lobe and grating lobe artifacts usually occur with strong reflectors in the near-field and appear at improper, off-axis locations.
- These artifactual echoes are most obvious within anechoic structures, such as breast cysts.

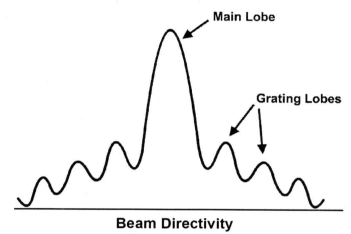

Beam Directivity

(Reprinted from Miele F: Ultrasound Physics and Instrumentation, 4th Ed., Miele Enterprises, 2006.)

7. Axial resolution artifact

- Failure to resolve two separate reflectors in the direction of the sound beam so closely spaced objects appear as one.
- Related to transducer frequency; spatial pulse length.

8. Lateral resolution artifact

- Failure to resolve two separate reflectors perpendicular to the sound beam.
- Primarily related to beamwidth and affected by focusing.

9. Slice thickness artifact

- "Fill-in" effect related to fact that the beamwidth is not razor thin.
- Can be a cause of false echoes within a cyst or mass from beam (volume) averaging.
- Occurs at region of poor elevational resolution.

10. Banding

- Focal band-like region of increased echogenicity corresponding to the level of the focal zone
- Related to the increased intensity of the sound beam at the focal zone

11. Speckle; Noise

- Appears as false echoes in tissue texture (granular appearance).
- Caused by the interference (constructive and destructive) of echoes from multiple scatterers.
- Acoustic speckle, clutter or "noise" produce weak amplitude echoes and can be related to excessive gain or electrical interference.
- Creates bright and dark spots on the image.
- Can affect apparent detail and contrast resolution.

12. Doppler Artifacts

- Excessive gain and too low filter setting can cause noise.
- High filter setting will reduce detection of low velocity blood flow.
- Too low of a PRF /velocity scale can cause aliasing.
- Spectral mirroring causes duplicate waveform on opposite side of baseline.
- If spectral or color Doppler angle is perpendicular to flow, no flow will be detected when flow is present.

13. Fremitus

- Color or power Doppler motion artifact produce from tissue vibration from the chest when the patient is asked to hum during scanning.
- Useful in establishing the boundaries of an attenuating breast mass, and differentiating a true mass from normal tissue. Normal structures will readily transmit the Doppler artifact.
  (See images in Examination Technique section.)

G. Quality Assurance - Phantoms

A variety of companies make multi-purpose monofilament and tissue-mimicking phantoms that allows the performance of a variety of quality assurance tests on breast ultrasound transducers.

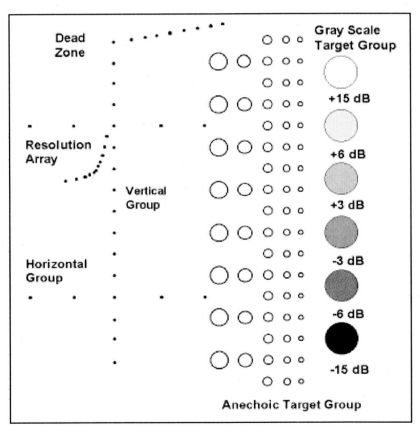

Schematic of ATS Multipurpose Phantom Model539
(Courtesy: ATS Laboratories, Inc., Bridgeport, CT)

Examples of parameters that can be tested include:

- Dead Zone
- Axial Resolution
- Lateral Resolution
- Focal Zone
- Vertical measurement calibration

- Image uniformity
- Sensitivity
- Cyst target delineation and measurement
- Grayscale and Displayed Dynamic Range
- Horizontal measurement calibration

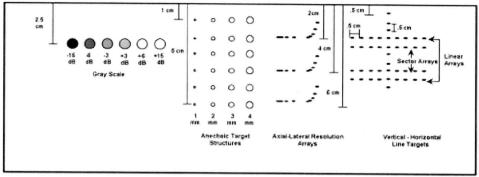

Schematic of ATS Model 550 Breast Scanning and Small Parts Phantom

Some manufacturers produce breast phantoms that contain cystic and solid tissue mimicking targets that allow the practitioner to learn and to refine skills necessary to perform ultrasound-guided aspirations or biopsies.

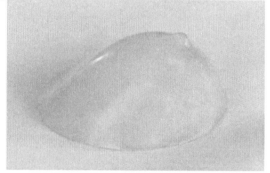

ATS Model BB-1 Breast Biopsy Phantom

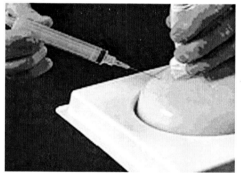

CIRS Model 052A Breast Needle Biopsy Phantom

• CHAPTER TWO •

Breast Sonography Examination

A. Clinical Role of Breast Sonography

1. Indications

AIUM /ACR Practice Guidelines cite the following as appropriate indications for breast sonography:
- Initial imaging technique to evaluate palpable mass in woman under age 30; and in pregnant or lactating woman
- Identification and characterization of palpable and nonpalpable abnormalities
- Evaluation and characterization of mammographic findings or other imaging exam (e.g., MRI)
- Evaluation of problems associated with breast implants
- Guidance during interventional procedures
- Treatment planning for radiation therapy

Additional or more specific indications for breast sonography include:
- Evaluation of the radiographic dense breast especially in high-risk patient
- Verification of suspected mass in area of asymmetric mammographic density
- Verification of location or presence of a mass seen on one x-ray view
- Breast evaluation when mammography is contraindicated or compromised (cases of trauma, irradiation, mastitis, male breast)
- Serial evaluation of a benign mass

2. Advantages

Advantages of sonography as a breast imaging modality include:
- Non-ionizing technique
- Painless
- Tomographic display without superimposition of structures
- Accurate differentiation between solid and cystic masses
- Relatively low cost examination
- Allows imaging close to chest wall
- Doppler capabilities allow detection of blood flow

3. Disadvantages-Limitations

Disadvantages or limitations of breast sonography include:
- Highly operator dependent
- Equipment quality dependent
- Limited ability to detect microcalcifications*
- Overlap in imaging features of some benign and malignant masses
- Artifacts and some normal structures (e.g., isolated fat lobule; costal cartilage; Cooper's ligament shadowing) can simulate pathology
- In the past, there has been a lack of standardization of technique and variability in the terminology used for the interpretation of findings. (The ACR has recently published a BI-RADS Ultrasound Lexicon.)

*AIUM and ACR Performance Guidelines state that although the efficacy of ultrasound as a screening study for occult masses is an area for research, at the current time, ultrasound is NOT indicated as a screening study for microcalcifications.

B. Patient and Examination Preparation

Before beginning a breast ultrasound examination, the sonographer should:

- Know the indication for and the scope of the examination requested
  (targeted vs. whole breast exam; unilateral vs. bilateral; follow-up exam; needle-guidance)
- Explain the procedure to the patient
- Obtain a pertinent clinical history including results of physical breast examination
- Obtain /Review pertinent correlative imaging tests *(e.g., prior mammogram, sonogram, MRI)*

1. Targeted vs. Whole Breast Examination

a. Targeted examination: (more common)
  - Limited to the area of mammographic concern
    (to further characterize findings so as to better assess the risk for malignancy; assign BI-RADS classification)
  - Limited to the area of clinical concern
    (e.g., in young, pregnant or lactating patient; or in patient with a palpable lump and a negative or equivocal mammogram)

Sonography's role in performing a targeted breast examination is to provide additional information to make a more specific diagnosis.

b. Whole breast (complete) examination - Indications include:
  - Breast secretions
  - High-risk patient with radiographic dense breasts
  - Search for satellite lesions in patient with known breast cancer
  - Silicone leakage associated with implant rupture
  - Search for primary lesion in patient with breast metastasis and a negative or equivocal mammogram
  - Follow-up of multiple known sonographic / mammographic masses
  - Patients who refuse mammography (radiation phobia)

2. Clinical History

Clinical and physical findings should be correlated with imaging findings. Some benign changes associated with trauma, infection, or irradiation can mimic malignancy. Clinical correlation is important before the interpreting physician assigns a risk level, renders a differential diagnosis, or makes management recommendations.

A pertinent patient clinical history should include:
- Current clinical symptoms
- Personal or family history of breast cancer
- Personal history of atypical duct hyperplasia
- Sites and findings regarding prior breast surgeries or aspirations
- History of breast infection, trauma, irradiation
- Atypical duct discharge
- Age, parity, and hormonal status (LMP; pregnant; hormone therapy)

3. Clinical – Physical Breast Examination

Visual findings assess:
- Symmetry and contour changes
- Skin thickening; discoloration; dimpling
- Nipple discharge; flattening; retraction
- Location of surgical scars
- Location of moles or other dermatologic conditions

Physical examination of a palpable mass can assess:
- Shape (round, oval, lobulated, irregular)
- Location relative to skin, nipple
- Consistency and compressibility (soft, firm, rubbery)
- Mobility (movable; fixed)

4. Mammographic Examination
Prior to the sonographic examination, the mammogram must be reviewed.
(See Chapter 4 on Mammographic and Sonographic Correlation)

C. Examination Technique

1. Patient Positioning

a. Supine Oblique (Contralateral Posterior Oblique) Position
A supine-oblique position is best suited for general breast scanning and, specifically, for evaluating the outer breast.

The patient is initially placed supine and then rolled into a contralateral posterior oblique position, elevating the side to be examined. A wedge-shaped sponge helps to support the patient's back and shoulder. The ipsilateral arm is extended near the head to better facilitate access to the axillary region and to help stabilize the breast tissues. This supine-oblique position allows even distribution of the breast tissue over the chest wall with central placement of the nipple.

The degree of obliquity can be changed to minimize breast thickness in the region being scanned. Greater degrees of obliquity are required for examining a mass in the outer, peripheral breast or when examining a large, pendulous breast.

Advantages of the supine-oblique position include:
- Minimizes breast thickness so tissues can be penetrated using a higher frequency transducer with better focusing characteristics.
- Flattens breast tissues and aligns tissue planes more parallel with the skin and transducer face, which reduces critical angle shadowing from Cooper's ligaments.

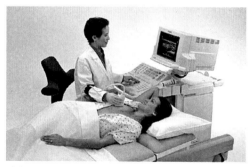

Contralateral posterior oblique (supine-oblique) positioning. (Courtesy: Philips Medical Systems)

b. Straight Supine Position
A straight supine position with the ipsilateral arm extended by head, optimizes examination of the medial breast by flattening tissues over the chest wall.

c. Other Positioning Options
For a palpable mass: Sometimes a mass can only be palpated in a specific position. The patient should initially be positioned in a manner that BEST facilitates palpation and scanning of the mass.

Sitting - Upright position: Upright scanning, and positioning the patient in a manner simulating the mammographic view, can allow better correlation of a lesion's location with the mammogram.

2. **Ergonomics**

    Attention to ergonomics is important for sonographer comfort and safety.

    • Raise the bed or stretcher, or sit at the level of the bed, so that the examination is conducted with the sonographer's shoulder and arm in a relaxed position.

    • Adjust the level and the angle of the display monitor to optimize viewing and to reduce neck strain.

    • Hold transducer securely at its base, instead of high on the cord.

    • The forearm may need to be lightly rested on the patient's torso for support.

    • Apply just enough transducer pressure to maintain good skin contact when not performing dynamic compression maneuvers.

3. **Grayscale Set-Up**

    For breast imaging, the echogenicity of breast tissues and masses are described in comparison to that of normal breast fat in accordance with ACR Lexicon descriptors. The gain settings and dynamic range should be adjusted so the echogenicity of fat is a medium (mid) level gray shade.

    The relative echogenicity of breast masses / tissues can be described as:

    Hypoechoic   =   less echogenic than fat
    Isoechoic   =   similar echogenicity as compared to fat
    Hyperechoic =   more echogenic than fat
    (Anechoic   =   echo-free; absence of internal echoes)

    Subtle degrees of hypoechogenicity of a mass are more discernable when the echogenicity is compared to fat, rather than to hyperechoic, fibroglandular tissue.

4. **Scan Planes**

    The region of a mass, or a specific breast quadrant, should be scanned in overlapping orthogonal planes: *(orthogonal planes are 90° apart)*

    • Longitudinal (Sagittal); Transverse
    • Radial; Antiradial

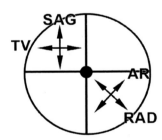

    Radial scans are oriented around the nipple like the "hands of a clock". Antiradial scans are perpendicular to the corresponding radial plane. The radial scan plane is best suited for evaluation of the major lactiferous ducts. Radial and antiradial scan planes help study the major ducts and smaller branching ducts. All solid masses should be scanned in radial and antiradial planes to check for subtle tumor projections that course toward the nipple, or branch outward in the breast.

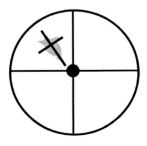

5. Echo-palpation

Echo-palpation allows real-time scanning during palpation for direct correlation of clinical and sonographic findings.

Methods:
- The palpable mass is immobilized between two fingers while scanning over the mass.
- The sonographer's finger is placed over the palpable mass; the transducer is placed over the finger, and then the finger is removed during real-time scanning to verify correlation.

6. Acoustic Standoff

Use of an acoustic standoff device or pad can improve imaging of superficial breast structures and masses by optimizing near field focusing and by reducing slice thickness artifacts. (Ample use of scanning gel can also provide an acoustic offset.)

In general, the thickness of the acoustic standoff pad should not exceed 1.0cm for transducers with an elevation focus of ≤ 1.5 cm. If a thicker standoff is used, the elevation focus can be shifted outside of the breast.

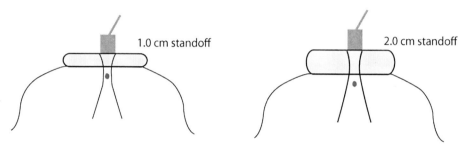

(Schematic reprinted with permission from SDMS/Pegasus Breast Ultrasound Exam Simulation CD, 2003)

When using a standoff pad, a reverberation artifact is commonly seen within the breast that is generated from strong specular reflection at the skin/standoff interface and the transducer/standoff interface.

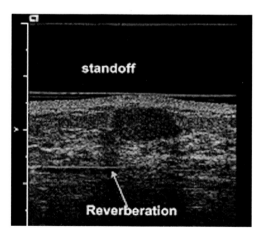

An acoustic standoff is less often needed with modern, high-frequency, breast ultrasound transducers with short-focal lengths, and for systems with compound imaging capabilities.

7. **Specialty Maneuvers For Examining Subareolar Structures**

Besides standard maneuvers, there are two specialty techniques recently described by Cindy Rapp, BS, RDMS and A.T. Stavros, MD that improve evaluation of subareolar tissues and ducts, as well as ducts existing the nipple. These methods are useful when the patient is in the supine or supine-oblique position.

Two-handed Peripheral Compression Technique
- Orient transducer radially along long axis of duct
- Place the nonscanning hand on the opposite side of breast by the subareolar tissues
- Press the transducer down along the breast tissue and slide distally to include the nipple, while applying pressure with the opposite hand

This maneuver brings the subareolar duct into a scan plane more parallel to the skin and also compresses the duct.

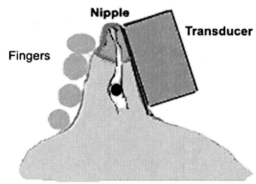

Two-handed Peripheral Compression Technique

Rolled-Nipple Technique
- Place the transducer at the edge of nipple in a radial plane parallel to the long axis of the duct
- Place the index finger of the nonscanning hand on the opposite side of the nipple from the transducer
- Apply light transducer pressure to force the nipple onto its side over the index finger

This maneuver allows the subareolar duct to be followed and imaged as it passes through the nipple, allowing demonstration of an intraductal mass.

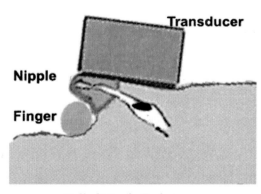

Rolled Nipple Technique

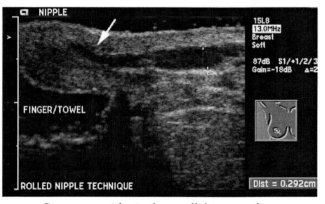

Sonogram with nipple parallel to transducer optimizing visualization of duct.

8. **Dynamic Compression**

Using variable transducer compression during the sonographic examination is useful for the following reasons:
- Decreases breast tissue thickness for better sound penetration
- Reduces critical angle shadowing from Cooper's ligaments by pushing normal breast tissues into a plane more parallel to the skin
- Reduces or eliminates false shadowing beneath a benign lesion or scar tissue (malignant shadowing persists)
- Assesses lesion compressibility
- Assesses lesion mobility and rotation
- Assesses movement of internal echoes of complicated cystic mass
- Assesses movement of echoes within a dilated duct

Drawbacks to using excessive transducer pressure over a mass include:
- Reduction in Doppler blood flow sensitivity since heavy compression can reduce or ablate blood flow within or around a mass
- Poorer margin delineation if transducer pressure compresses adjacent, tissue against the mass
- Poorer delineation of superficial lesions because of near field artifacts and poor focusing (In these cases, a lighter transducer pressure is recommended.)

9. **Variable Transducer Angulation**

Angling the transducer from multiple directions allows better assessment of the margin characteristics of a mass, and of the completeness of the capsule.

This is accomplished by:
- Rocking transducer from end-to-end (heel-toe maneuver)
- Rocking transducer from side-to-side
- Rotating transducer
- Scanning coronally

The margin of a mass is best seen when the sound beam is perpendicular to the interface, thereby maximizing specular reflection back to the transducer. Enlarging the field-of-view helps in the evaluation of margin characteristics.

10. **Vocal Fremitus**

Fremitus refers to the "thrill" of the chest wall when the patient vocalizes.

To help differentiate abnormal from normal breast tissue, power Doppler can be applied to the region of a breast mass while having the patient "hum". The chest vibration creates a Doppler signal, termed fremitus. During this maneuver, normal breast tissue vibrates and generates a color or power Doppler signal. The region of a "true" mass will be void of this Doppler effect. The area of "drop-out" indicates the boundaries of the mass.

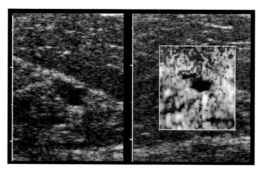

Practical uses of vocal fremitus include:
- Better delineation the borders of a poorly-defined mass from surrounding tissues
- Differentiation of a fat lobule from a true solid mass
- Differentiation of multifocal from unifocal disease
- Differentiation of artifactual shadowing from true shadowing

11. Image Documentation

Ultrasound images of important findings should be recorded on a retrievable and reviewable image storage format, which may include digital PACS archival.

Image labeling should include: (ACR Practice Guidlines)
- The facility name and location
- Examination date
- Patient's name; identification number and / or date of birth
- Anatomic location of the area scanned or of mass location using an acceptable annotation method:
  - breast side (right or left)
  - quadrant notation
  - clock notation or labeled diagram of breast
  - distance from nipple
  - transducer orientation (scan plane)
- Appropriate mass measurement with 1 set of images obtained without calipers. The maximal dimensions of a mass should be recorded in a minimum of 2 scan planes.
- Sonographer's or sonologist's initials or identification.

For interventional procedures, the relationship of the needle to the mass should be documented. (e.g., pre-fire and post-fire biopsy image documentation).

12. Mass Measurement

The ACR states that maximal dimensions of a mass should be documented in at least 2 scan planes (orthogonal planes recommended.) The 2 maximal ultrasound measurements correlate best with mammographic dimensions.

Obtaining three dimensions permits calculation of mass volume for serial follow-up, which is helpful when assessing a tumor's response to chemotherapy, and for assessing length vs. height ratios. The longest dimension of the mass is sought and measured as the mass' length (or longitudinal axis). The dimension perpendicular to this axis is the short axis measurement. The third measurement is recorded in the orthogonal plane. A "mean diameter" can then be generated, which may be easier to use when following mass size over a time interval.

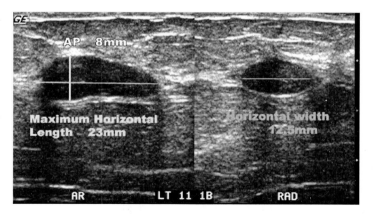

The 2 maximal dimensions of a mass on a sonogram correlate best with the mammographic measurements. The "short-axis" of a mass is not typically shown on a mammogram. This is especially true if a mass is oval (ellipsoid) in shape or very compressible.

Note:
When measuring suspicious lesions, areas of duct extension, branch pattern, and the echogenic rim of tumor infiltration should be included on an image, since these features are components of the tumor.

13. Annotation Methods

a. Side / Quadrant Annotation
    Breast quadrants and related segments are annotated as follows:

RUOQ	Right Upper Outer Quadrant	LUOQ	Left Upper Outer Quadrant
RUIQ	Right Upper Inner Quadrant	LUIQ	Left Upper Inner Quadrant
RLOQ	Right Lower Outer Quadrant	LLOQ	Left Lower Outer Quadrant
RLIQ	Right Lower Inner Quadrant	LLIQ	Left Lower Inner Quadrant

SA   Subareolar   AX   Axilla

b. Clock-Face Method
    Representative images of the breast can be recorded of each breast quadrant and identified by clock-face position. A radial scan plane extends in a direction similar to the "hands of a clock" with the nipple centrally located.

    The location of a breast mass can be indicated by its clock-face position.

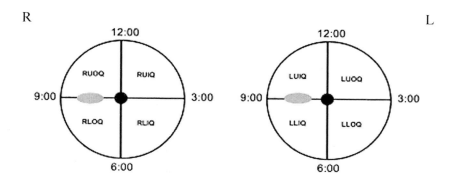

A mass located at the 9:00 position in the right breast is lateral to the nipple.
A mass located at the 9:00 position in the left breast is medial to the nipple.

c. Distance from Nipple Annotation
    When annotating mass location using the clock-face position or a labeled diagram on the image, the distance of the mass from the nipple should be noted.

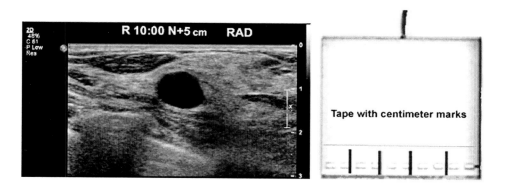

This image is annotated R 10:00 N+5 cm RAD indicating the lesion is 5 cm from the nipple at the 10:00 position in the right breast with the transducer in the radial scan plane.

If the nipple is seen on the same ultrasound image as the mass, calipers can be placed for distance measurements. Most transducers are 3.5 to 5 cm in length and can be used to help estimate the distance between the nipple and a mass. Placing a piece of tape with centimeter marks along the side of the transducer can assist measurement.

d.   123-ABC Annotation Methods

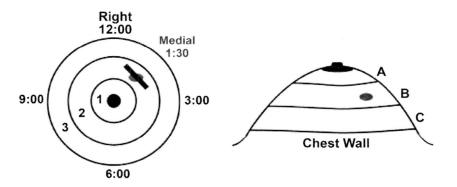

RT 1:30 2B AR
(Schematic reprinted with permission from SDMS/Pegasus Breast Ultrasound Exam Simulation CD, 2003)

Some facilities use the "1-2-3" and "ABC" labeling methods to denote the location of a breast mass. These methods can be combined with the breast side, clock-face position, and scan plane notation to provide a more specific description of mass location and transducer orientation.

"123 method" denotes the approximate distance of the mass from the nipple.
  The breast is divided into 3 equal width rings around the areola:
    1 = near the nipple/areola
    2 = mid distance from nipple
    3 = periphery of the breast

"ABC method" denotes the approximate depth of the lesion in the breast:
    A = near the skin
    B = mid depth (mammary zone)
    C = near the chest wall

The diagram shows a mass that is located in the right (RT) breast; at the 1:30 clock position; located mid distance from the nipple (2); located mid depth in the breast (B); and scanned in the antiradial (AR) plane.

The scan plane is not always noted with the 123-ABC method.

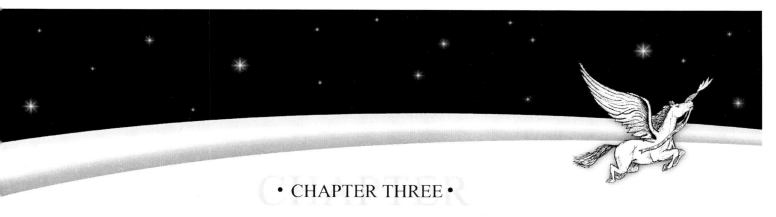

• CHAPTER THREE •

Breast Anatomy and Development

A. Breast Development

The development of the mammary glands begins in the 4th week of embryonic life (6th menstrual week). Paired regions of ectodermal thickening occur at intervals along bilateral mammary ridges or "milk lines." These milklines extend from each axilla to the inguinal regions. One pair, along the upper one-third of the milk lines, persists to eventually form the breasts. During the remainder of fetal life, epithelial cells proliferate and gradually form buds and cords of cells that project into the subcutaneous tissues. During the last three months of gestation, secondary buds eventually canalized to form rudimentary lactiferous ducts. By birth, little more than the main ducts have developed in both males and females.

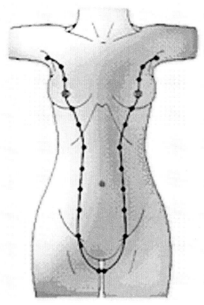

Bilateral milklines

The newborn male or female may show mild physiologic prominence of the breast tissue (ducts) due to the residual effects of maternal hormones. These effects subside as hormonal levels return to normal.

The breasts of males and females are generally similar until puberty, when estrogen and other hormones initiate breast development in the female. During adolescence, the breast lobules form within the female. The male breast remains in an underdeveloped state.

With each menstrual cycle, the female breast undergoes proliferative and involutional changes. Further maturation of the breast occurs with pregnancy and lactation.

B. Developmental Anomalies - Variants

1. **Unilateral Early Ripening (Premature Thelarche)**
   Between the ages of 6-8 years, the glandular tissue of one breast may start to develop before the other. This presents as a tender discoid lump beneath the areola. Usually by age 9 or by puberty, both breasts are of similar size. Sonographically, the developing glandular tissue appears as a hypoechoic, subareolar nodular region.

   Unilateral early ripening of a breast should not be mistaken for a mass and does not require biopsy. Excision will remove vital glandular tissue and prevent further breast development (surgical cause of amazia).

2. **Bilateral Early Breast Development – Precocious Puberty**
   Bilateral early breast development can be associated with precocious puberty. Causes include estrogen-secreting ovarian or adrenal tumor, or changes within the hypothalamus or pituitary glands.

3. **Congenital nipple flattening or inversion**
   Nipple flattening or inversion can be congenital, especially if bilateral.
   New findings are suspicious for pathology.

4. **Polythelia**
   Polythelia is the presence of accessory (supernumerary) nipples. This is the most common developmental anomaly and affects both males and females. An accessory nipple is most often located just inferior to the breast, but can develop anywhere along the milk lines.

5. **Polymastia**
   Polymastia is the presence of accessory (supernumerary) breasts. A fully formed accessory breast with nipple/areolar tissue is rare. Accessory mammary tissue (without the nipple/areola) is more common and often forms in the axillary region.

6. **Athelia** is the absence of a nipple.

7. **Amastia** is the absence of development of a breast and nipple.

8. **Amazia** is the absence of development of breast tissue. This can occur secondary to excessive radiation exposure or from surgical excision.

C. Breast Anatomy

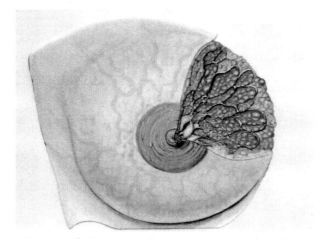

Reprinted: Carnation Company, Los Angeles, 1966

1. External Anatomy

The adult female breasts are paired, domed-shaped, modified apocrine sweat glands. The mammary glands are located anterior to the muscles overlying the 2nd- 6th ribs, and extend from the sternal edge to mid axillary line.

  a. Skin

  The skin of the breast is composed of the epidermis and dermis. The skin is thickest at the base of the breast. Pores along the surface of the skin indicate the locations of sweat glands, sebaceous (oil) glands, and hair follicles.

  b. Nipple / Areola Complex

  The nipple is a round, fibromuscular papilla projecting from the center of the breast. Small excretory ducts exit the surface of the nipple and drain the lactiferous ducts.

  The areola is a region of smooth, circular, pigmented skin that encircles the nipple. The areola contains numerous sebaceous glands (Montgomery's glands) that appear as small nodules under the skin. These glands release a fatty substance that protects the nipple during lactation.

2. Internal Anatomy

The mature female breast is composed of varying mixtures of fat, glandular, and fibrous connective tissues, besides blood vessels, lymphatics, and nerves. The glandular tissue of the breast is enclosed between the superficial and deep layers of the superficial fascia. The breast parenchyma contains the functional glandular elements of the breast and their supporting stroma. Extension of glandular tissue into the axilla is called the axillary tail of Spence. Breast fat is found beneath the skin, beneath the glandular tissue, and fills the spaces between the lobes. The subcutaneous fat does not extend beneath the nipple.

  a. Functional Glandular Tissues

  The adult female breast is composed of 15-20 lobes that contain the functional, epithelial elements of the breast. The overlapping lobes are arranged in a radial fashion around the nipple. The greatest amount of glandular tissue resides within the upper outer quadrant of the breast.

  The function of the breast is to produce milk during lactation. Each lobe contains numerous lobules, which are drained by small branching ducts that unite to form a main lacteriferous duct (segmental duct; lobar duct). This main duct widens just below the nipple at the lactiferous sinus (ampulla). The lactiferous sinus serves as a reservoir for milk or secretions that accumulate beneath the areola. If some of the main ducts join beneath the areola, a lesser number of excretory ducts will exit through the nipple.

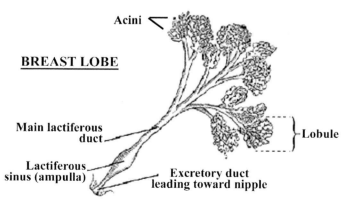

(Schematic reprinted with permission from SDMS/Pegasus Breast Ultrasound Exam Simulation CD, 2003)

The functional unit of the breast is the terminal duct lobular unit (TDLU). The TDLU is composed of an extralobular terminal duct and a lobule. The lobule contains an intralobular terminal duct that drains multiple (30-50) tiny blind-ended ductules. These ductules correspond to tiny the saccular, milk-producing glands of the breast called the acini. The acini fully form during pregnancy and lactation, and then involute to a variable degree following cessation of lactation.

The number and size of TDLUs vary with the patient's age and hormonal status. Rapid proliferation of the lobules occurs during early reproductive life, during the postovulatory phase of the menstrual cycle, and during pregnancy and lactation. Regression or atrophy of the lobules is more pronounced following pregnancy/lactation and menopause.

The TDLU is an important anatomic structure since it is the site of origin of most breast pathologies.

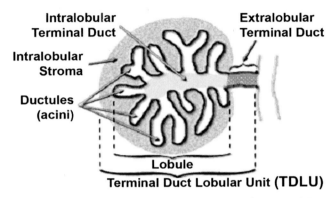

(Schematics reprinted with permission: SDMS/Pegasus Breast Ultrasound Exam Simulation CD, 2003)

The ducts are lined by specialized cells and are bounded by the basement membrane. The inner lining of the ducts is composed of epithelial cells. Beneath the epithelium is a layer of more widely-spaced myoepithelial cells that lie by the basement membrane of the duct. The myoepithelial cells contain contractile fibers that aid in the transport of milk from the acini and ducts.

In the nonlactational breast, the lumen of the ducts may contain variable amounts of fluid, protein, and cellular debris.

b. Stromal Tissue

Stromal tissues are the supportive elements of the breast and consist of fat (adipose) and fibrous connective tissues. Loose intralobular stroma surrounds the small ductal structures within the lobule. This stroma gives the lobule its shape and definition. The extensive capillary network of the intralobular stroma allows the exchange of hormones into, and secretions out of, the lobule. This specialized stroma contains lymphocytes, histiocytes, plasma cells, and mast cells. Dense extralobular (interlobular) stroma lies between the lobes and lobules and supports the larger ductal structures. The breast is also supported by dense connective tissue septa, called Cooper's ligaments. These suspensory ligaments extend from the deep layer of the superficial fascia to the skin and separate fat lobules and lobes.

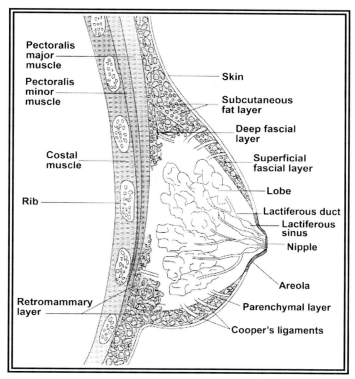

Anatomic components of the female breast. (Reprinted with permission: Carr-Hoefer C: Breast, In Diagnostic Medical Sonography, Kawamura D (ed), Philadelphia, Lippincott, 1997)

5. **Vascular Anatomy**

a. Arterial Supply

The main arterial supply to the breast is from branches of the lateral thoracic artery (external mammary artery) and from perforating branches of the internal mammary artery (internal thoracic artery). The lateral thoracic artery arises from the axillary artery distal to the thoracoacromial artery. It passes inferiorly along the lateral border of the breast and gives off branches that supply the lateral breast. The internal mammary artery arises from the subclavian artery and descends behind the costal cartilages of the upper ribs near the sternum. Perforating branches supply blood to the medial breast.

Smaller amounts of blood are supplied by perforating branches of the intercostal artery and the pectoral branch of the thoracoacrominal artery. The intercostal branches help perfuse the lower breast, whereas the thoracoacrominal branches help perfuse the upper breast.

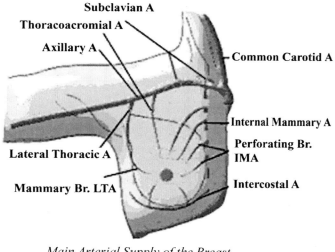

Main Arterial Supply of the Breast

b. Venous Drainage
Blood is drained from the breast by superficial and deep venous systems. Venous anastomoses occur in a circular pattern beneath the areola. The superficial and deep veins communicate throughout the mammary tissue.

The superficial veins course beneath the superficial fascia. Communication can exist between the superficial veins of both breasts.

The deep veins travel alongside the arteries and drain into the internal mammary, axillary, subclavian, and the intercostal veins. The veins are routes of hematogenous metastases from carcinomas. Intercostal veins anastomose with vertebral veins and can provide a pathway for bone metastases.

6. **Nerves**
Nerves are found within the skin and glandular tissue of the breast. Branches of the intercostal (thoracic) nerves primarily innervate the breast. Branches of the supraclavicular nerve also innervate the superior and lateral aspect of the breast.

7. **Lymphatic Anatomy**
Lymphatic channels originate in the interlobular connective tissue and the walls of the lactiferous ducts. Lymph flow begins deep within the breast. The direction of lymph flow is toward the subareolar plexus where the intramammary and subdermal lymphatics anastomose under the areola. Flow through the superficial channels is directed outward toward the lymphatic chains that drain the breast.

Intramammary lymph nodes are found within the breast. Lymphatic drainage closely follows the path of the veins and empties into the axillary, internal mammary, and intercostal chains of lymph nodes. A small amount of lymph can drain from channels that cross the mid chest to the contralateral breast. Some drainage can extend to the supraclavicular nodes, or to the diaphragmatic nodes. Intramammary lymph nodes are found within the breast, especially in the upper outer quadrant.

a. Axillary Lymph Nodes
Most of the lymph ($\geq$ 75%) drains into the axillary lymph nodes.

There are 30-40 lymph nodes along the axillary chain, which are subdivided into anatomic groups.

Anatomic Classification – Axillary Lymph Node Chain	
External mammary	Nodes along the lateral thoracic vessels
Subscapular	Nodes along the subscapular vessels
Axillary	Nodes along the lateral part of the axillary vessels
Central	Nodes along the medial part of the axillary vessels; embedded in fat in the center of the axilla
Subclavicular (infraclavicular)	Nodes along the subclavian vessels medial to the origin of the thoracoacromial artery
Interpectoral (Rotter's)	Nodes between the pectoral major and minor muscles; along the pectoral branch of the thoracoacromial artery

The axillary lymph nodes are the most common site for lymphatic metastasis from breast cancer. For surgical and staging purposes, the axillary lymph nodes are divided into three levels relative to the pectoralis minor muscle.

Surgical Classification – Axillary Lymph Nodes		
Level I	Low axilla	Nodes lateral to pectoralis minor muscle
Level II	Mid axilla	Nodes deep to the pectoralis minor muscle; or Nodes located between the medial and lateral borders of the pectoralis minor muscle *(This later classification includes Rotter's nodes)*
Level III	High axilla	Nodes medial to the pectoralis minor muscle *(apical – subclavicular nodes)*

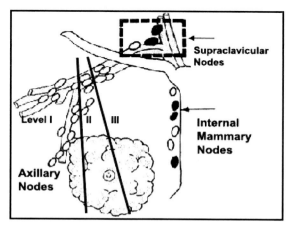

Regional lymph nodes of the breast.

b. Internal Mammary Lymph Nodes
   The internal mammary lymph nodes (parasternal nodes) follow the path of the internal mammary arteries and veins. These nodes lie within the 2nd-4th intercostal spaces just lateral to each side of the sternum. Lymph drains to the internal mammary nodes via channels that penetrate through the chest wall into the intercostals spaces.

   (Medially located cancers may metastasize to the internal mammary nodes. These nodes also provide collateral drainage for lateral tumors when axillary nodes are obstructed. Ultrasound is helpful in assessing parasternal lymphadenopathy since these nodes are not detectable on a mammogram or by clinical palpation.)

c. Supraclavicular Lymph Nodes
   The supraclavicular lymph nodes lie in the supraclavicular fossa near the internal jugular and subclavian veins. Lymph must pass through the deep jugular or subclavian nodal chains to reach the supraclavicular nodes.

D. Sonographic Anatomy
   Many of the anatomic components of the breast are demonstrated with high-resolution breast sonography. The appearance of normal female breast varies depending on the amount of fat, connective, and glandular tissues in the scanning plane.

1. Grayscale set-up
   For breast imaging, the system gain and dynamic range should be adjusted so that echogenicity of fat appears as a medium-level gray shade. The echogenicities of tissues and masses are reported in comparison to that of normal breast fat.

Relative Echogenicities of Normal Breast Tissues			
Isoechoic/Nearly Isoechoic	**Hyperechoic**	**Hypoechoic**	**Anechoic**
Fat	Skin	Nipple	Duct secretion
Epithelium (TDLU)	Cooper's Ligaments	Blood	Blood in vessel
Loose stromal fibrous tissue (surrounding ducts of lobule; periductal)	Dense interlobular stromal fibrous tissue	Milk in duct	Milk in duct

- *Normal fat is used as the reference tissue to compare echogenicities.*
- *Dense interlobular fibrous stroma will appear more echogenic than loose intralobular or periductal stromal fibrous tissue.*

> cyst fluid< blood < muscle < **fat** ≤ glandular tissue < fibrous tissue/C.Lig < calcification

2. **Tomographic Sonographic Anatomy**
   Sonography allows sectional evaluation of the breast, one "slice" at a time, from the skin to the chest wall. Levels identified include:
   - Skin layer – Nipple/areola
   - Subcutaneous fat layer
   - Mammary layer (parenchyma; fibroglandular tissue)
   - Retromammary fat layer
   - Pectoralis Muscle layers (deep to the breast)
   - Ribs / Intercostal muscles
   - Pleura-Lung

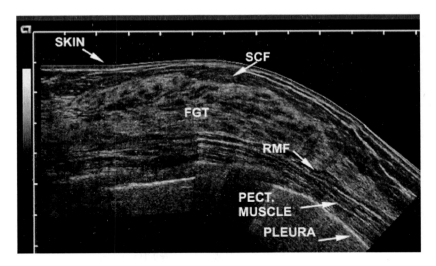

Main Breast Layers	Zones
Subcutaneous	Pre-mammary
Mammary (Parenchymal)	Mammary
Retromammary	Retromammary

   a. Skin Layer
      The skin is echogenic relative to the subcutaneous fat. The skin layer is composed of epidermis and dermis and is usually ≤ 2mm in thickness. The skin can be thicker in the inferior breast and the areolar region.

Scanning Tips:

Use of an acoustic standoff allows better focusing at the skin level and better demonstration of the skin contour. When scanning through a standoff pad, the skin appears as two thin, hyperechoic lines encasing a medium-level band of echoes (the dermis). The two highly reflective lines are from the offset/epidermis and the dermis/fat interfaces. Extra scan gel also serves as an acoustic standoff. Transducer compression can affect skin thickness.

Changes in skin contour and thickness may indicate neoplastic, traumatic, post irradiation, or inflammatory changes at or below the skin level.

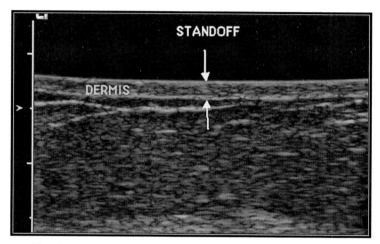

Skin layer seen well when scanned though acoustic standoff.

b. Nipple – Areola Complex

The nipple usually displays a homogeneous texture of low-to-medium level internal echoes. The areola is thicker than the surrounding skin of the breast.

Acoustic shadowing is often generated from the nipple/areola region due to:
*   Attenuative connective tissues within the nipple
*   Irregular skin contour causing poor skin contact or air gaps between the transducer and the skin/areola/nipple

Scanning Tips to better evaluate the subareolar region include:
*   Use of ample acoustic gel and transducer pressure to compress the nipple and to eliminate trapped air pockets
*   Placement of the transducer along side of the areola and angling under the nipple
*   Performance of specialty maneuvers: 2-handed peripheral compression; rolled-nipple technique
*   Spatial compound imaging
*   Use of acoustic offset (standoff pad, extra gel) to evaluate the nipple

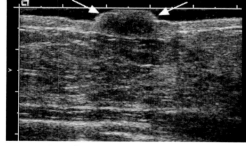

Nipple-Areola complex

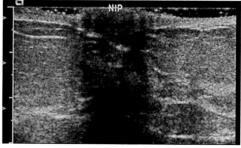

Nipple shadowing

c. Subcutaneous Fat Layer
The subcutaneous layer lies between the skin and mammary layer. It is primarily composed of fat lobules enclosed by connective tissue septa. Blood vessels, lymphatics and nerves also reside within this superficial layer. Subcutaneous fat does not extend beneath the nipple.

Gain settings should be adjusted so fat displays a medium-level gray-shade. Fat lobules appear oval in one plane and elongated in the orthogonal plane.

Cooper's ligaments are best seen in the subcutaneous layer and appear as thin, hyperechoic, curvilinear bands that extend around the fat lobules toward the skin. Critical angle shadowing can occur from oblique sound incidence to these connective bands.

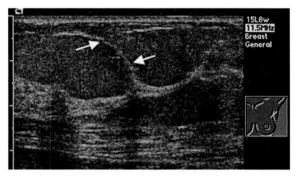

Hyperechoic Cooper's ligaments best seen in subcutaneous fat layer.

Scanning tips to reduce Cooper's ligament shadowing include:
*   Increase transducer pressure to flatten the ligaments
*   Angle transducer so scan plane is more perpendicular to ligament

d. Mammary Layer
The mammary layer lies between the subcutaneous and retromammary fat layers and contains the fibroglandular tissue (parenchyma) of the breast. (Although the TDLUs are primarily located within the mammary layer, there are instances when a TDLU may extend into either fat layer.)

The sonographic appearance of the mammary layer (zone) varies between individuals, and significantly changes with regards to the female's age and hormonal status (pregnancy, lactation, menopause). Fibroglandular tissue is typically hyperechoic when compared to fat, primarily due to the dense fibrous stromal elements. When sonographically visible, glandular tissues (TDLUs; ductal structures), along with loose stromal fibrous tissue within the mammary zone tend to be more isoechoic to fat.

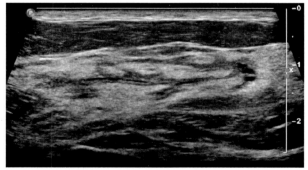

Relative to fat, fibrous tissue of the mammary layer is hyperechoic as compared to the nearly isoechoic periductal glandular tissue.

Fluid-filled lactiferous ducts can be visualized within this breast layer. The main lobar ducts are best seen on radial scans. Ducts increase in size as they approach the nipple. Generally, ducts measure ≤2mm but can be larger at the lactiferous sinus and during pregnancy or lactation. Doppler differentiates fluid-filled ducts from arteries or veins.

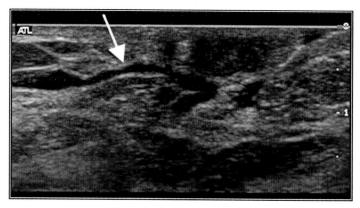

Fluid-filled subareolar lactiferous ducts.
SDMS/Pegasus Breast Ultrasound Exam Simulation CD, 2003

The superficial and deep layers of the superficial fascia (premammary and retromammary fascia) encase the mammary layer and are occasionally seen as thin, hyperechoic lines when the sound beam is directed perpendicular to the fascial planes.

e. Retromammary Fat Layer
The retromammary fat layer separates the mammary layer from the pectoralis muscle and contains adipose tissue and connective fascia. This layer is thinner and contains smaller fat lobules than the subcutaneous fat layer. The TCG and overall gain settings should be adjusted so both fat layers are of similar echogenicity.

The retromammary space lies between the deep layer of the superficial fascia and the deep pectoral fascia. This space allows the breast to move freely over the muscle layer.

f. Muscle Layers
Two-thirds of the breast tissue lies anterior to the pectoralis major muscle. This large muscle runs obliquely from the mid sternum and medial half of the clavicle to the greater tubercle of the humerus. Sonographic visualization of this muscle is important since it verifies that the sound beam has fully penetrated the breast tissue.

Muscles:
Pectoralis Major

Pectoralis Minor

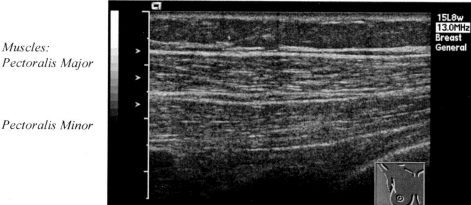

The pectoralis minor muscle is located beneath the upper, outer portion of the pectoralis major muscle. The pectoralis minor muscle is an important landmark for determining the surgical levels of the axillary lymph nodes.

On a sonogram, the pectoral fascia overlying the pectoralis major muscle produces a thin, hyperechoic band of echoes. The muscles are hypoechoic and contain hyperechoic linear striations along the long axis of the muscle. The chest wall includes the serratus anterior muscle, ribs, and the intercostal muscles. The serratus anterior muscle lies posterior to the lower outer quadrant of the breast. The intercostal muscles are demonstrated between the ribs, and beneath the pectoralis muscle.

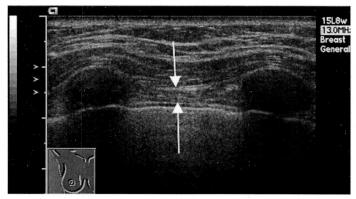

Intercostal muscles seen between hypoechoic costal cartilages.
SDMS/Pegasus Breast Ultrasound Exam Simulation CD, 2003

g. Ribs, Pleura
The bony ribs attenuate the sound beam causing acoustic shadowing. More medially, the costal cartilages are less attenuative. On sagittal scans, the costal cartilages appear as regularly-spaced, oval, hypoechoic structures. Care must be taken not to mistake a rib cartilage for a breast mass.

Deep to the intercostal muscle and ribs is the pleura of the lung. Since sound does not penetrate the air-filled lung, the pleural interface is the deepest structure identified on a breast sonogram. The highly reflective lung interface produces a hyperechogenic band of echoes.

h. Lymph Nodes
Occasionally, normal lymph nodes are seen within the mammary zone and the subcutaneous fat layers. Most intramammary lymph nodes are located in the posterior, upper outer quadrant. Intramammary nodes typically measure less than 1cm. Normal lymph nodes may also be seen in the axillary regions and often exceed 1cm in size. Internal mammary lymph nodes are not usually detected by on a sonogram unless enlarged.

The sonographic features of normal lymph nodes include:
*   Oval or reniform shape with smooth margins
*   Hypoechoic outer cortex
*   Hyperechoic fatty hilum (with Doppler flow)

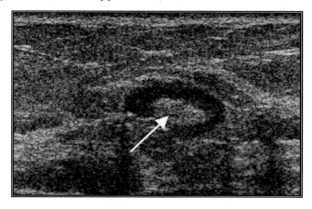

44

E. Breast Physiology

The design and function of the breast is to produce milk. Although the breast does not produce hormones, the breast tissues respond to a variety of hormones produced by the ovaries, hypothalamus and pituitary glands, placenta, thyroid, and pancreas.

The two most prominent hormones active in breast physiology are:
- Estrogen- responsible for ductal proliferation
- Progesterone - responsible for lobular proliferation and growth

Prolactin is another important hormone that is present during late pregnancy and lactation.

1. Menstrual Cycle Changes

Cyclic changes occur in the breast with each menstrual cycle that causes an increase in glandular tissue.

During the first part of the menstrual cycle, estrogen stimulates epithelial proliferation and enlargement of the larger ductal structures within the breast.

With ovulation, progesterone levels rise. Progesterone stimulates growth of the lobules and the terminal ductules following ovulation. These changes, along with increased blood flow and interstitial fluid retention, causes physical symptoms of premenstrual breast tenderness, fullness and nodularity.

The onset of menses occurs with declining progesterone levels. Changes within the lobular units begin to regress and involute. Some changes persist.

2. Pregnancy and Lactational Changes

Major Hormonal Influence on the Breast During Pregnancy and Lactation		
Hormone	**Influence on breast**	**Produced by**
Estrogen	Stimulates growth and division of the ducts	Ovary
Progesterone	Stimulates increase in size and number of the lobules and maturation of acini	Ovary, placenta
Prolactin-inhibiting factor	Prevents the release of prolactin until milk production is needed after childbirth	Hypothalamus
Prolactin	Stimulates acini to produce milk	Anterior pituitary gland
Oxytocin	Initiates contraction of ducts for flow of milk during lactation	Posterior pituitary gland
Other hormones:	Placental lactogen; HCG	Placenta

Changes in the breast are seen within several weeks of conception. Epithelial cells and ducts proliferate, increasing the size and number of the TDLUs. The acini become fully formed within the lobules in anticipation for milk production. After birth, prolactin levels increase, acini undergo secretary changes, and milk is produced. After lactation ends, these structures begin to involute and regress to a variable degree.

3. Involutional Changes and Menopause

Involution of glandular tissues occurs following cessation of lactation, ovarian ablation (by surgical removal, radiation therapy, or chemotherapy) or with natural menopause. Very few mature lobules normally persist past menopause. The sharp decline in hormone production leads to atrophic changes of the lobules, which may be replaced by fat or sclerosis. Use of hormone replacement therapy (HRT) can retard involutional changes. Combined estrogen-progesterone HRT may even cause postmenopausal persistence or development of mature lobules.

After menopause, the relative amount of breast fat increases as glandular-epithelial structures atrophy.

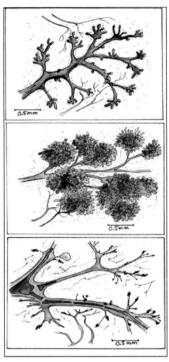

Hormonal Changes Affecting Lobules
www.mammary.nih.gov

F. Normal Sonographic Variations Related to Age-Hormonal Status

1. Prepubertal Breast

The prepubertal breast is small and fatty. A small, hypoechoic-to-echogenic region of glandular tissue beneath the nipple represents early development of the parenchyma.

2. Adolescent Breast

Following puberty, the adolescent breast becomes increasingly glandular and the amount of fat decreases. Sonographically, this parenchyma has a very fine, uniform, weakly-echogenic texture (similar to fat). The surrounding fat layers may be too thin to be visualized on the sonogram.

3. Adult Breast

The adult breast has the greatest range of appearances. The young nulliparous female breast is densely glandular with little internal or surrounding fat. With an increase in stromal tissue, the fibroglandular tissue becomes more hyperechoic. With advancing age and parity, more fat is deposited in the fat layers, as well as in the mammary zone.

4. Pregnancy and Lactation

During pregnancy / lactation, the glandular tissue dramatically expands and compresses the surrounding fat. The glandular tissue is less reflective than fibrous tissue and appears isoechoic or mildly hyperechoic relative to fat. This gives the breast a fine, "ground-glass" appearance. With milk production, the ducts dilate and contain anechoic or hypoechoic fluid.

5. Postmenopausal Breast

Menopausal changes cause atrophy of the parenchymal structures and a relative increased deposition of breast fat. Residual fibroglandular tissue may persist mainly beneath the nipple and upper outer breast quadrant. On a sonogram, the hyperechoic Cooper's ligaments are easily seen encasing the fat lobules. Older nulliparous women, or those on hormone replacement therapy, may retain greater amounts of glandular tissue.

Pegasus Lectures, Inc.

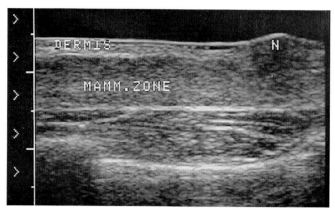

Young, nulliparous breast with a homogeneous, isoechoic
glandular pattern with minimal, if any surrounding fat.

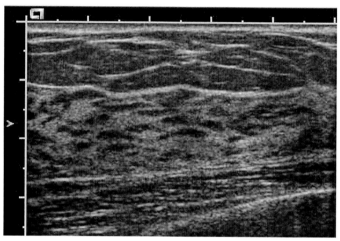

Adult breast showing mixed pattern of fibroglandular tissue.
The glandular, ductal elements are relatively isoechoic to fat.
The fibrous stromal tissue is hyperechoic compared to fat.

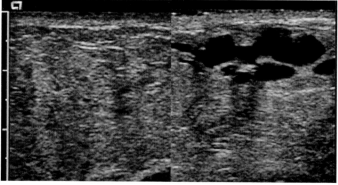

Lactational breast showing expansive glandular tissue and duct dilatation.

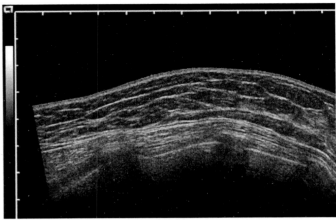

Postmenopausal atrophy with fatty replacement of the glandular tissue.

• CHAPTER FOUR •

Mammographic & Sonographic Correlation

A. Mammographic Examination
Mammography is performed for screening or for diagnostic purposes.

1. Screening Mammography
- Purpose is to detect breast cancer in an asymptomatic patient.
- Allows detection of a greater number of early cancers, stage 0 (in situ) and stage 1, which improves survival.
- Currently the best imaging modality for the detection of suspicious microcalcifications, which are the earliest sign of an occult malignancy.
- Detection of calcifications/masses is best in the fat-replaced breast.
- Detection of pathology is significantly reduced in dense breast tissue.
- Standard screening views include bilateral medioloateral oblique (MLO) and craniocaudal (CC) projections.
- ACR Practice Guidelines recommend yearly screening mammograms for asymptomatic women age 40 years or older.

2. Diagnostic (Problem-Solving) Mammography
- Evaluatation of clinical symptom such as lump or thickening, nipple discharge, skin changes, etc.
- Further examination of an abnormality found on a screening exam.
- Typically requires additional views besides standard views.

B. Mammographic Views – Image Orientation
The mammographic image represents a summation of breast tissues compressed between the x-ray and compression plates.

1. Standard Mammographic Views

Mediolateral oblique (MLO) view
- Superimposition of breast tissue from superomedial to inferolateral.
- Projection parallel to the pectoralis muscle.
- C-arm of mammographic unit is angled 30^0-60^0 (generally at 45^0).
- Side marker is placed by the axilla / upper outer breast.
- Best view for showing the upper outer quadrant, axillary tail, and pectoralis major muscle. (Most breast cancers occur in the UOQ and can be visualized in this view.)
- Generally estimates mass location as superior or inferior in the breast (with some variation).

Craniocaudal (CC) view
- Superimposes superior over inferior breast tissue.
- Side marker is placed by the lateral (outer) breast.
- Shows truer location of the mass as medial or lateral relative to the nipple. Best view for showing subareolar, central, and medial breast.
- Helps detect posteromedial tumors missed on the MLO view.

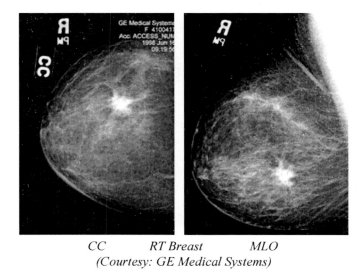

CC   RT Breast   MLO
(Courtesy: GE Medical Systems)

From these standards views, the location of a mass can be approximated. The posterior nipple line is a reference point for determining mass location.

a. Ultrasound lesion localization based on MLO and CC views
A mass located in the medial breast on the CC view will actually lie slightly higher in the breast than the location indicated on the MLO view.

A mass located in the lateral breast on the CC view will actually lie lower in the breast than that indicated on the MLO view. Peripheral lesions show a greater degree of shift in location.

(acronym MULD: medial up; lateral down)

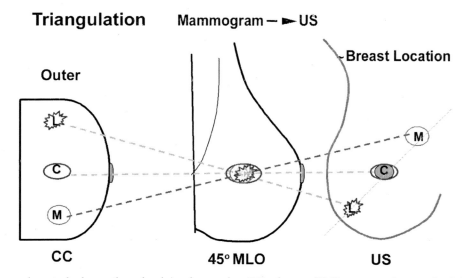

A mass located along the nipple axis on the CC view will lie approximate the MLO location for sonomammographic correlation.

Pegasus Lectures, Inc.

b. Some additional (non-standard) mammographic views
   90⁰ (True/Straight) Lateral view:
   - Superimposes medial over lateral tissue.
   - Performed to better delineate questionable, superimposed tissues from that of a true mass.
   - Shows true position of a mass or calcifications superior or inferior to the nipple (which is helpful for pre-surgical localization).
   - Used for biopsy and localization procedures.

   Spot compression views

   Magnification views

   Exaggerated craniocaudal views

C. Mammographic-Sonographic Tissue Comparison

The sonographer should understand the correlation between the density of tissues seen on a mammogram with the echogenicity of similar tissues seen on the sonogram.

Tissue Type	Mammographic Density	Sonographic Echogenicity
Fat	Medium gray Fat density; Radiolucent	Reference tissue; Gain set to display fat as medium gray shade
Parenchyma (Fibroglandular Tissue)	Radiodensity greater than fat Water density May be radiopaque	Typically hyperechoic or mixed pattern depending on amount of fibrous elements. Ductal tissues less echogenic than fibrous tissue and nearly isoechoic to fat.
Fluid-filled Duct Blood Vessel	Radiodensity greater than fat Water-density	Centrally anechoic; hypoechoic
Cyst	Radiodensity greater than fat May be radiopaque Water-density	Anechoic; Hypoechoic (particulate echoes)
Lymph Node	Radiodense (water density) cortex Radiolucent (fat density) hilum	Hypoechoic cortex Hyperechoic (fatty) hilum
Solid Mass Benign/Malignant	Radiodensity greater than fat Water-density May be radiopaque	Isoechoic; mild-to-markedly hypoechoic
Calcification	Radiopaque	Markedly hyperechoic
Pectoralis Muscle	Higher density than fat Radiopaque	Striated hyperechoic/hypoechoic pattern

The types of tissue densities seen on a mammogram are fat, water, air, and calcium. Both cystic and solid masses are "water density" on a mammogram, which is more dense than fat. Mammographically detected masses can be described as being of high, equal, or low density (as compared to an equal volume of fibroglandular tissue), or as fat-density. Malignant masses are usually very dense for their size.

Fat-containing masses are typically benign and include post-traumatic oil cysts, lipomas, and galactoceles. Hamartomas also contain fat components.

Unlike mammography, sonography can easily differentiate cysts from solid masses, in part, because of their differences in echogenicity and attenuation characteristics.

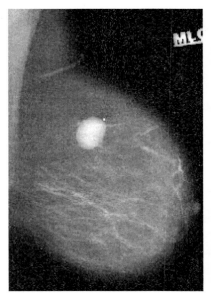 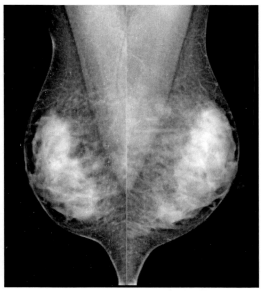

Mammogram: High-density mass is easily seen in the fat-replaced breast.

Water density fibroglandular tissue can potentially obscure a water-density cyst or solid mass. (Courtesy: GE Medical Systems)

On a mammogram, detection of masses and calcifications is best in the fat-replaced breast. Low and high-density masses will be easily contrasted against the translucent gray background of fat. Dense breast tissue can obscure detection of an isodense, water-density mass.

On a sonogram, detection of masses is best when contrasted against a background of hyperechoic, fibroglandular tissue. Small isoechoic masses can be missed in the fatty breast.

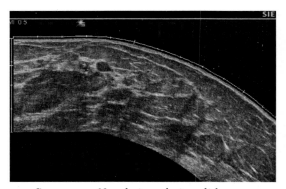 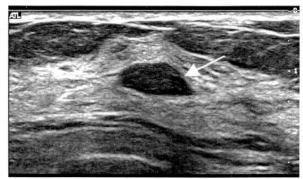

Sonogram: Nearly isoechoic solid mass in primarily-fatty breast

Solid mass is more readily seen when contrasted against a background of hyperechoic fibrous tissue.

D. Sonographic-Mammographic Correlation

The correlating mammogram must be reviewed by the sonographer and interpreting physician prior to the sonographic examination and before interpretation of findings.

Correlation of sonographic and mammographic features of a mass should include:
- Size, shape, margins
- Location in breast
- Density of surrounding tissues

Correlation is particularly important in a patient with multiple breast masses to verify that the abnormality seen on the mammogram correlates with the abnormality seen on the ultrasound.

It is important not to confuse an incidental finding on the sonogram as the cause of a mammographic mass if the size, shape, location, and the density of the surrounding tissues do not correlate.

Note: Supine or supine-oblique positioning flattens the breast tissue over the chest wall. This can cause the location of a breast mass to appear deeper on the sonogram than that seen on the mammogram. A mammogram is performed upright with tissues compressed and pulled away from the chest wall. Rescanning the patient in an upright position may be necessary to better correlate the sonographic and mammographic locations of a mass.

Tissue - Lesion Depth

MAMM

US

9 cm

3 cm

CC positioning -
Tissue compressed and
pulled away from chest wall

US - Tissue compressed
and pushed toward chest
wall from transducer pressure.

The CC view on the mammogram is generally comparable to the transverse view on the sonogram. Because of the variable degree of obliquity, it is more difficult to correlate the location of a mass on the MLO view with the sonographic longitudinal view.

US Simulation of CC view

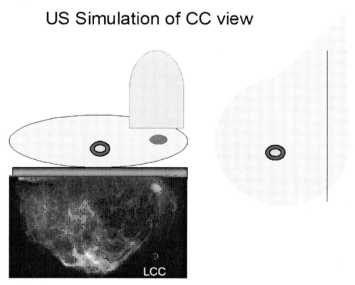

LCC

On a mammogram, a solid or cystic "water-density" mass that is surrounded by other water-density tissues (e.g., fibroglandular tissue, capsule of the mass) can generate a "combined mass-effect" that is larger on the mammogram than the actual size of the mass on the sonogram. For better sono-mammographic correlation, the sonographer should include measurements on the sonogram of tissues surrounding the mass that would explain the mammographic findings in addition to measuring the mass.

• CHAPTER FIVE •

Benign vs. Malignant Features
Descriptive Terminology

A. Mammographic Imaging Assessment BI-RADS

The BI-RADS® classification system was developed by ACR to promote reporting consistency in the mammographic interpretation of breast disease. Assessment categories are based on the risk for malignancy. Specific recommendations for patient management are based on risk level.

American College of Radiology (ACR) Breast Imaging Reporting and Data System BI-RADS® Mammographic Assessment Categories			
Category	**Classification**	**Risk of Malignancy**	**Recommendation**
0	Incomplete		Need additional imaging
1	Negative		Routine F/U for age
2	Benign Finding	0 %	Routine F/U for age
3	Probably Benign	≤ 2 %	Short-term F/U
4	Suspicious Abnormality	3- 94 %	Consider tissue sampling
5	Highly suggestive of malignancy	≥ 95%	Tissue sampling

BI-RADS® category 4 can be further subdivided as:
  4A: Low suspicion
  4B: Indeterminate
  4C: Moderate suspicion

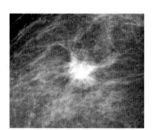

Mammographic features suspicious for malignancy include:
* Spiculated, irregular, or ill-defined mass
  (Spiculation is the most specific sign of malignancy =BI-RADS 5)
* Clustered calcifications (>5 calcifications/cm^3) or other suspicious branching or linear pattern
* Focal architectural distortion
* (Enlarging non-cystic mass)
* Secondary signs (nipple retraction, skin thickening, enlarged dense nodes etc.)

BI-RADS® Category 0 indicates mammographic assessment is "incomplete" and additional imaging, such as additional mammographic views or sonography, is indicated before a final risk classification is assigned. After sonography is performed, the risk classification can be revised.

The ultrasound characteristics of a mass should be described using accepted terminology. The ACR has recently released an ultrasound BI-RADS lexicon form to promote standardization in the description and classification of breast masses seen by sonography.

B. ACR–BI-RADS®–US Lexicon Classification Form

For each of the following categories, select the term that best describes the dominant lesion feature. Wherever possible, definitions and descriptions used in BI-RADS® for mammography will be applied to ultrasound. This form is for data collection and does not constitute a written Ultrasound report

1. **Masses: A <u>mass</u> occupies space and should be seen in two different projections.**

Shape *(select one)*		Description
☐	Oval	Elliptical or egg-shaped (may include 2 or 3 undulations, i.e. "gently lobulated" or "macrolobulated)
☐	Round	Spherical, ball-shaped, circular, or globular
☐	Irregular	Neither round nor oval in shape

Orientation *(select one)*		Description
☐	Parallel	Long axis of lesion parallels the skin line ("wider than tall" or horizontal)
☐	Not Parallel	No long axis, or axis not oriented along the skin line ("taller than wide" or vertical)

Margin *(select one)*		Description
☐	Circumscribed	A margin that is well defined or sharp, with an abrupt transition between the lesion and surrounding tissue
☐	Not Circumscribed*	The mass has one or more of the following features: indistinct, angular, microlobulated or spiculated
☐	Indistinct	No clear demarcation between a mass and its surrounding tissue
☐	Angular	Some or all of the margin has sharp corners, often forming acute angles
☐	Microlobulated	Short cycle undulations impart a scalloped appearance to the margin of the mass
☐	Spiculated	Margin is formed or characterized by sharp lines projecting from the mass

Lesion Boundary *(select one)*		Description
☐	Abrupt interface	The sharp demarcation between the lesion and surrounding tissue can be imperceptible or a distinct well-defined echogenic rim of any thickness.
☐	Echogenic Halo	No sharp demarcation between the mass and surrounding tissue, which is bridged by an echogenic transition zone.

Echo Pattern (select one)	Description
☐ Anechoic	Without internal echoes
☐ Hyperechoic	Having increased echogenicity relative to fat or equal to fibroglandular tissue
☐ Complex	Mass contains both anechoic (cystic) and echogenic (solid) components
☐ Hypoechoic	Defined relative to fat; masses are characterized by low-level echoes throughout (e.g. appearance of a complicated cyst or fibroadenoma)
☐ Isoechoic	Having the same echogenicity as fat (a complicated cyst or fibroadenoma may be isoechoic or hypoechoic)

Posterior Acoustic Features (select one)	Description
☐ No posterior acoustic features	No posterior shadowing or enhancement
☐ Enhancement	Increased posterior echoes
☐ Shadowing	Decreased posterior echoes; excluding edge shadows
☐ Combined pattern	More than one pattern of posterior attenuation, both shadowing and enhancement

Note: Irregular is used as descriptor of shape rather than margin

Surrounding Tissue	Description

Identifiable effect (select all that apply)

☐ Duct changes	Abnormal caliber and/or arborization
☐ Cooper's ligament changes	Straightening or thickening of Cooper's ligaments
☐ Edema	Increased echogenicity of surrounding tissue: reticulated pattern of angular, hypoechoic lines
☐ Architectural distortion	Disruption of normal anatomic planes
☐ Skin thickening	Focal or diffuse skin thickening-Normal skin is 2 mm or less in thickness except in the periareolar area and lower breasts
☐ Skin retraction/ irregularity	Skin surface is concave or ill-defined, and appears pulled in

2. **Calcifications: Calcifications are poorly characterized with ultrasound but can be recognized particularly in a mass.**

Calcifications	Description

If present (select all that apply)

☐ Macrocalcifications	Greater than or equal to 0.5 mm in size
☐ Microcalcifications out of mass	Echogenic foci that do not occupy the entire acoustic beam and do not shadow. Less than 0.5 mm in diameter.
☐ Microcalcifications in mass	Embedded in a mass, microcalcifications are well depicted. The punctate, hyperechoic foci will be conspicuous in a hypoechoic mass

3. **Special Cases: Special cases are those with a unique diagnosis or finding.**

Special Cases (select all that apply)	Description
☐ Clustered microcysts	A cluster of tiny anechoic foci, each smaller than 2-3 mm in diameter with thin (less than 0.5 mm) intervening septations and no discrete solid components
☐ Complicated cysts	Most commonly characterized by homogeneous low-level internal echoes. Complicated cysts may also have, fluid-fluid, or fluid-debris levels that may shift with changes in patient's position.
☐ Mass in or on skin	These masses are clinically apparent and may include sebaceous or epidermal inclusion cysts, keloids, moles and neurofibromas.
☐ Foreign body	May include marker clips, coil, wire, catheter sleeves, silicone, and metal or glass related to trauma.
☐ Lymph nodes - intramammary	Lymph nodes resemble small kidneys with an echogenic hilus and hypoechoic-surrounding cortex. Found in the breast, including axilla
☐ Lymph nodes - axillary	Lymph nodes resemble small kidneys with an echogenic hilus and hypoechoic-surrounding cortex. Found in the breast, including axilla

4. **Vascularity**

Vascularity *(select one)*

- ☐ Not present or assessed
- ☐ Present in lesion
- ☐ Present immediately adjacent to lesion
- ☐ Diffusely increased vascularity in surrounding tissue

5. **Assessment Category** *(select one)*

Assessment Category (select one)	Description
☐ Category 0 – Incomplete: Need additional imaging evaluation	Additional imaging evaluation needed before final assessment

Final Assessment

☐ Category 1 – Negative	No lesion found (routine follow-up)
☐ Category 2 –Benign finding	No malignant features; e.g. cyst (routine follow-up or age, clinical management)
☐ Category 3 – Probably benign finding	Low probability of malignancy e.g. fibroadenoma (short interval follow-up,).
☐ Category 4 – Suspicious abnormality	Intermediate probability of malignancy, (biopsy should be considered)
☐ Category 5 – Highly suggestive of malignancy	High probability of malignancy, (appropriate action should be taken)
☐ Category 6 – Known cancer	Biopsy proven malignancy, prior to definitive of therapy (appropriate action should be taken)

Printed with permission: American College of Radiology; Copyright© 2003

Pegasus Lectures, Inc.

C. Primary and Secondary Diagnostic Features

Sonographically, breast disease is divided into two groups:
- Mass
- Disorders without a discrete mass
  (architectural distortion)

A "mass" occupies space and has 3-dimensions. Orthogonal scans planes outline the dimensions of a true mass.

The morphological features of a mass are divided into:

1. **Primary Features: Describe specific characteristics of the mass**
   - Size
   - Shape
   - Orientation
   - Margin clarity and regularity
   - Margin / Border thickness
   - Echogenicity
   - Homogenicity
   - Attenuation Effects

2. **Secondary Features: Describe the effects of the mass on surrounding tissues; or changes in tissues in response to the mass**
   - Interruption of tissue planes
   - Duct dilatation; tumor extension
   - Echogenicity of the subcutaneous fat
   - Thickening, straightening, retraction of Cooper's ligaments
   - Lymphatic dilatation; edema
   - Skin changes
   - Lymph node enlargement

3. **Dynamic Tests:**
   - Compressibility
   - Mobility
   - Doppler features

D. Sonographic Features – Cystic Masses

Sonographic Characteristic – Benign Simple Breast Cyst	
Diagnostic Features*	• Round, oval shape • Smooth, thin walls • Absent internal echoes • Posterior sound enhancement • Bilateral thin edge shadowing
Additional Features	• Dynamic tests: Compressibility / Mobility • Absent internal Doppler signal

When all diagnostic features are present, the diagnostic accuracy approaches 100%.

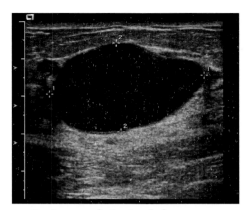

Benign anechoic simple breast cyst.

Complicated Cysts – Complex Fluid Masses	
Diagnostic Features	• Diffuse low-level internal echoes • Fluid-debris level • Fluid-fluid; Fluid-fat level • Thin septations • Thick septations • Circumferential isoechoic wall thickening • Eccentric wall thickening • Intramural nodule

Many complicated cysts are related to benign fibrocystic change.

Complex mass features more suspicious for malignancy:
•   Thick, isoehoic septations
•   Irregular, eccentric wall thickening
•   Intramural nodule

Complex/Complicated cyst features more worrisome for inflammation:
•   Isoechoic wall thickening
•   Fluid-debris levels (may be present)
•   Hyperemia of cyst wall seen with Doppler

Cyst aspiration / biopsy allows a definitive diagnosis.

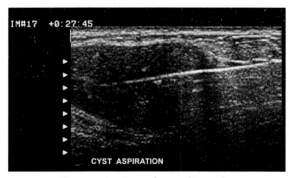

Cyst aspiration of complicated cyst.

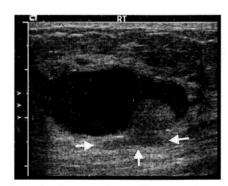

Complex intracystic papillary carcinoma in situ.

Pegasus Lectures, Inc.

E. Benign Sonographic Features - Solid Masses

The following two tables are based on criteria reported by Dr. A.T. Stavros.

Benign Sonographic Findings - Solid Mass/Nodule *(Stavros et al)*	
Benign Finding	**Description**
Absent malignant findings	Benign imaging features are sought after all malignant features have been excluded.
Marked hyperechogenicity	Pure, uniform hyperechoic tissue (cannot contain hypoechoic areas larger than normal ducts or TDLUs ≤ 4mm) *Typically associated with benign fibrous stromal tissue; focal ridge of fibroglandular tissue that presents as a clinical and/or a mammographic pseudomass.*
Mass features:	
Ellipsoid; Wider-than-Tall	Oval mass that measures greater in its horizontal dimensions than in AP dimension. Horizontal orientation = parallel to skin
2-3 gentle macrolobulations	Gently-curving, smoothly lobulated contours
Thin echogenic pseudocapsule	Pseudocapsule of compressed tissue surrounding the mass *Represents slow-growing, non-infiltrative leading edge of mass; Capsule must be complete on all surfaces*
(Smooth, well-circumscribed)	**(All features)**

A thin echogenic pseudocapsule must accompany a mass with an ellipsoid shape or with 2-3 gentle lobulations.

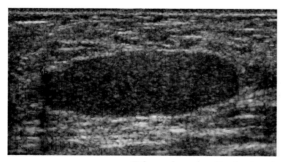 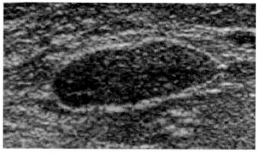

Fibroadeomas displaying benign sonographic features.

F. Malignant Sonographic Features – Solid Masses

Individual Malignant Sonographic Features - Solid Mass *(Stavros et al)*	
Malignant Finding	**Description**
Spiculation - Correlates to mammographic spiculation - Highest PPV for invasive cancer	Alternating hypoechoic / hyperechoic straight lines that radiate out perpendicularly from the surface of the mass *- hypoechoic relative to echogenic fibrous tissue* *- hyperechoic relative to surrounding fat* **Thick, echogenic halo = variant of spiculation** *(Represents infiltrative margin of mass)*
Angular margins	Irregular, jagged contour; can be acute / obtuse / 90⁰ angles *(Form at points of least resistance to tumor growth, such as at the base of Cooper's ligaments.)*
Taller-than-wide	AP dimension greater than horizontal dimensions *(Feature of small cancers growing within a vertically oriented TDLU; Can indicate growth across tissue planes)*
Acoustic shadowing	Shadowing behind all or part of the mass *(Typically related to the degree of desmoplasia, reactive fibrosis)*
Hypoechogenicity	Central part of mass is markedly hypoechoic as compared to fat *(Related to tumor cellularity and composition)*
Microcalcification	Tiny, nonshadowing, punctate hyperechoic foci best seen within a hypoechoic mass *(Lie within DCIS component of tumor)*
Duct extension	Tumor extension from the surface of the mass into or around a single duct leading toward the nipple *(Intraductal tumor; Best seen on radial scans)*
Branch pattern	Tumor extension from the surface of the mass into smaller ducts leading away from the nipple *(Intraductal tumor; Best seen on radial and antiradial scan planes in the region of the mass)*
Microlobulation	Multiple small surface lobulations (often ≤ 2mm) *(Can represent fingers of invasive tumor, intraductal components, or enlarged cancerized lobules)*
(Disruption of tissue planes)	

The presence of any single malignant feature excludes a mass from a benign BI-RADS classification. Most malignant masses show multiple malignant findings, which raises the level of suspicion. Imaging features are influenced by tumor morphology, growth rate, and the body's response to the presence of the cancer. Cancers can range in appearance from spiculated-to-circumscribed or show a combination of finding.

Malignant Imaging Features:

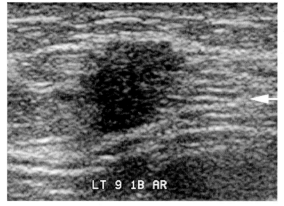

Spiculation.
(Courtesy: Cindy Rapp, BS, RDMS)

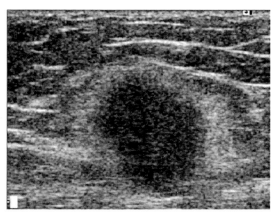

Thick echogenic halo; Taller-than wide;
Marked hypoechogenicity
(Courtesy: B.Fornage, MD)

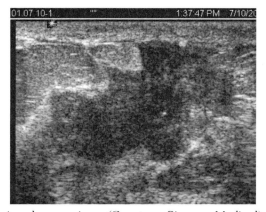

Angular margins.   (Courtesy: Siemens Medical)

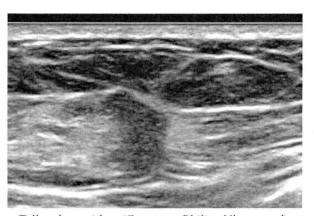

Taller-than-wide.   (Courtesy: Philips Ultrasound)

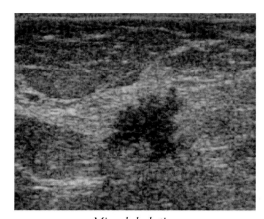

Microlobulation.
Marked hypoechogenicity
(Courtesy: Cindy Rapp)

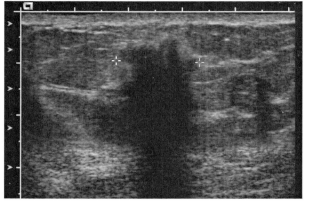

Acoustic Shadowing.

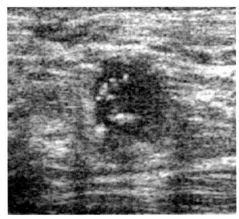

Microcalcifications.

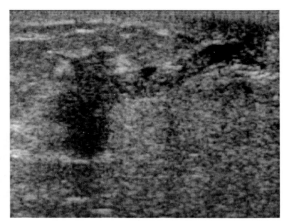

Duct extension toward the nipple.

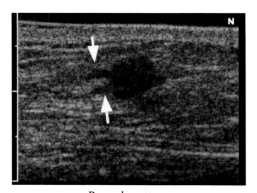

Branch pattern.
(Selected images reprinted with permission from SDMS/Pegasus Breast Ultrasound Exam Simulation CD, 2003)

Using Dr. Stavros' criteria, sonographic characteristics of solid masses that show less specificity in differentiating benign from malignant masses are:
- Homogeneous vs. heterogeneous echo pattern
  (in part, because calcifications were described as a separate entity from heterogenicity)
- Isoechogenicity or mild hypoechogenicity
- Normal sound transmission or posterior enhancement

Approach for sonographic evaluation of solid breast masses: (Stavros)
1. First evaluate for any individual malignant finding
2. If malignant findings are present, then the mass qualifies for either a BI-RADS 4 (a,b) or BI-RADS 5 classification. Biopsy is indicated.
3. If NO malignant findings are identified, search for benign sonographic features.
4. If benign sonographic findings ARE present, the findings are classified as either BI-RADS 2 or BI-RADS 3 ($\leq$ 2% risk for malignancy). Patient management choices for BI-RADS 3 include: short-term follow-up in 6 months or biopsy.
5. If benign sonographic findings are not detected, the mass is classified as BI-RADS 4(a) and biopsy is warranted.

Modified Breast Imaging Reporting And Data System (BI-RADS) Ultrasound Risk Categories*			
BI-RADS Category	Classification	Risk for Malignancy	Recommendation for Patient Management*
1	Normal	0	Clinical lump follow-up and return to screening
2	Benign finding	0	Clinical lump follow-up and return to screening
	Probably benign	≤ 2%	Patient choice: short-term follow-up or biopsy
4a	Mildly Suspicious	> 2% and < 50%	Biopsy
4b	Moderately Suspicious	> 50% and < 90%	Biopsy
5	Highly suspicious for malignancy	≥ 90%	Biopsy

*Generally suggested management, not rigid requirement
(Adapted from: Stavros AT. Breast Ultrasound. Philadelphia, Lippencott Williams & Wilkins, 2004, p.3)

Other common diagnostic criteria noted in the literature for the evaluation of solid breast masses include:

Benign vs. Malignant Solid Mass	
Benign Characteristics	Malignant Characteristics
• Round, oval shape • Well-defined, circumscribed margin • Orientation parallel to skin • Homogeneous texture • Acoustic enhancement	• Irregular shape • Poorly-defined, indistinct margin • Orientation non-parallel to skin • Heterogeneous texture • Central shadowing

Dr. Christopher Merritt, TJUH

Overview of Ultrasound Characteristics

In the literature, there are multiple ways to describe the features of breast masses. The following tables provide an overview of features.

Note: Some benign breast masses display malignant imaging features. Also, malignant masses display some benign features. Because of this overlap in findings, biopsy is recommended for a mass with even one suspicious finding.

Sharpness of Margins	Benign Features	Malignant Features
Clarity of margin delineation	• Well-defined • Well-circumscribed	• Ill-defined • Ill-distinct; In-distinct
Demarcation between mass and surrounding tissues	Non-infiltrative pattern: Indicates mass is displacing rather than infiltrating surrounding tissues. Sharp demarcation of mass from adjacent tissue.	Infiltrative growth pattern: Indicates invasion into adjacent tissue or host response. (Dx. Pitfall: benign traumatic or inflammatory changes)

On a mammogram, a well-circumscribed mass will demonstrate a thin radiolucent fat halo that represents the compressed tissue border. This is a benign feature.

Contour of Margins	Benign Features	Malignant Features
External shape or surface characteristics	• Smoothly circumscribed • Regular • 2-3 macrolobulations (Gently lobulated)	• Spiculated • Angular • Microlobulated • Indistinct

Border Thickness and Echogenicity	Benign Features	Malignant Features
	• Thin, echogenic pseudocapsule	• Thick, echogenic halo
	- Represents non-invasive leading edge of a slow-growing solid mass. (Rim of compressed tissue.) - Cyst may show a thin, imperceptible wall.	Infiltrative zone between mass and surrounding tissues. - Unresolved spiculation - Host-response - Peritumoral edema

Careful scanning is required when evaluating for a thick echogenic halo. Scanning tangentially though an echogenic halo my mimic benign hyperechogenicity. Scanning throughout the entire malignant lesion should reveal a central hypoechoic nidus.

Shape	Benign Features	Malignant Features
	• Round (especially if related to a cyst) • Oval; ellipsoid	• Irregular (although some cancers may be round or oval)

Orientation	Benign Features	Malignant Features
Relationship of long axis of mass to skin	• Long axis parallel to skin (Horizontal; Wider-than-tall)	• Non-parallel • Perpendicular to skin (Vertical; Taller-than-wide)
	Indicates non-invasive growth between normal tissue planes. Slow-growing, softer mass is more deformable by surrounding tissues.	Can indicate growth across tissue planes. Feature of small cancer (≤ 1.5cm) as grows within a vertically-oriented TDLU.

Echogenicity	Benign Features	Malignant Features
Refers to brightness of echoes within a breast mass or tissue, as compared to fat.	• Marked hyperechogenicity (e.g.,benign stromal tissue) • Anechoic (cyst)	• Marked hypoechogenicity (most worrisome)

Hypoechoic   *(less echogenic than fat)*
Isoechoic   *(echogenicity similar to that of fat - medium gray shade)*
Hyperechoic   *(more echogenic than fat)*

Echo Texture	Benign Features	Malignant Features
Echo pattern reflects composition and cellularity of mass	Homogeneous = Uniform distribution and intensity of internal echoes	Heterogeneous = Nonuniform distribution and intensity of internal echoes (hypoechoic+hyperechoic)

Both benign and malignant masses can show textural inhomogenicity. Benign causes can include fibrosis, sclerosis, degeneration, and calcification.

Effects on Distal Echoes	Benign Features	Malignant Features
Attenuation effects	• Enhancement (such as with simple cyst)	• Shadowing Typically related to the degree of fibroelastic response

Note: Not all cancers shadow. Hypercellular or necrotic cancers can show distal enhancement. Some benign masses may show shadowing, especially with scarring or fibrosis.

Compressibility Mobility	Benign Features	Malignant Features
Degree of deformability and movement of a mass from manual or transducer pressure	• Compressible and mobile (especially, non-tense fluid mass, fat lobule, lipoma, hamartoma)	• Noncompressible and fixed (associated with invasive cancer with fibrous response) (However, some highly cellular cancers may show some mild compressibility.)

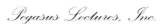

Vascularity	Benign Features	Malignant Features
Refers to the distribution and number of peripheral and intratumoral vessels; patterns of tissue vascularity; arterial or venous flow.	• Benign masses generally shows less internal blood flow than cancers. • Absent blood flow within cyst or fluid-filled mass • Hilar flow within lymph node • Increased blood flow associated with inflammation	• Neoangiogenesis associated with increased number of peripheral and internal vessels. Increased vessel tortuosity. • May show higher PSV • PI/RI values not considered reliable enough to differentiate cancer from benign.

Internal blood flow verifies the solid nature of a mass. Blood-flow differentiates vessels from ducts. Doppler findings are often reported as absent, increased, or decreased compared to adjacent tissues and not specifically used to differentiate benign from malignant solid masses.

Calcifications	Benign Features	Malignant Features
	• Macrocalcifications > 0.5mm	• Microcalcifications < 0.5mm
Note: US has limited ability to detect microcalcifications. Mammography is the best modality to image microcalcifications.	Rim calcification, and macrocalcifications are typically benign. Larger calcifications cause acoustic shadowing. *(Most microcalcifications are benign; often related to FCC such as milk of calcium cysts)*	Do not shadow since smaller than the beamwidth. US detection of these tiny, nonshadowing, hyperechoic foci are best seen within a hypoechoic mass or in a distended duct.

Effects on Fibrous Planes	Benign Features	Malignant Features
	• Cyst or solid mass cause displacement or compression of surrounding tissues • No interruption of tissue planes	• Disruption / interruption of tissue planes • Thickening / straightening of Cooper's ligaments; retraction of skin/nipple
	(Note: Benign inflammatory or traumatic changes can disrupt or distort affected tissues.)	• SC fat shows increase echogenicity with invasion • Skin invasion causes thickening, ↑↓ echogenicity • Pectoral invasion shows fixation to chest wall

Effects on Ducts	Benign Features	Malignant Features
Duct dilatation can be related to increased secretions; obstruction or tumor	• Generally < 2-3mm - Larger at lactiferous sinus - Taper within breast core	• Extension of tumor from mass into ducts • Intraductal tumor - (DICS, papillary CA)
	Normal dilatation with pregnancy and lactation	• Localized duct dilation • Duct irregularity • Wall thickening

Benign disorders associated with duct dilatation include ductal ectasia/periductal mastitis, FCC, intraductal papillary lesion.

Pegasus Lectures, Inc.

Nipple Discharge	Benign Features	Malignant Features
	Non-worrisome findings: • Expressible only • Bilateral • Multiple Duct Orifices • Milky or greenish color Most common pathologies - Intraductal Papilloma (most common cause of discharge; often bloody) - FCC (2nd most common) (green, milky, yellowish) - Periductal mastitis-Duct ectasia - Hyperprolactemia (prolactin-induced secretions): Bilateral; milky, multiple ducts - Idiopathic	Worrisome findings: • Spontaneous • Unilateral • Single duct orifice • Bloody; clear or serosanguinous Most common pathologies: - Papilloma (main benign cause of bloody discharge) - Papillary carcinoma - Carcinoma

Lymph nodes	Benign Features	Malignant Features
	• Oval, reniform shape • Circumscribed, smooth margins (thin, echogenic capsule) • Hypoechoic outer cortex • Hyperechoic fatty hilum • Doppler flow within hilum through single hilar artery Intramammary nodes usually ≤ 1cm Axillary nodes usually ≤ 2.5cm	• Rounded, lobulated, irregular shape • Enlargement • Displacement or loss of echogenic fatty hilum • Marked hypoechogenicity • Heterogeneous cortical echogenicity • Ill-distinct borders or irregular shape • Increased cortical and transcapsular blood flow

Skin Thickening	Benign Features	Malignant Features
	• Normal ≤ 2 mm	• Increased thickness • Altered, ↑ echogenicity • Dilated lymph channels
	Benign causes, skin thickening: • Trauma; Inflammation; Irradiation; Heart failure; Dermatologic condition; Nephrotic syndrome	Cancer related causes • Lymphatic obstruction • Direct invasion • Metastatic disease • Lymphoma • Inflammatory cancer

Notes:
- Benign processes with imaging features that can mimic carcinoma include:
  - Fat necrosis
  - Radiation changes
  - Sclerosing adenosis
  - Diabetic fibrosis
  - Scar
  - Radial scar
  - Granular cell tumor
  - Hyalinized fibroadenoma

- Abscesses and hematomas can show irregular margins and disrupt tissue planes. These entities may mimic cancer on a mammogram.

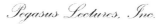

- Circumscribed cancers that may mimic benign tumors include:
  - High-grade invasive ductal   - Medullary
  - Colloid   - Papillary
  - Intracystic   - Phyllodes
  - Lymphoma   - Metastasis

- Not all cancers shadow and some show sound enhancement.

- Microcalcifications occur with both benign and malignant disease. However, microcalcifications in a hypoechoic solid mass are suspicious for malignancy.

• CHAPTER SIX •

Benign Breast Changes and Pathology

A. Fibrocystic Change

Fibrocystic change (FCC) is the most common diffuse breast disorder. This condition is not a disease, but represents a variety of relatively normal benign breast alterations induced by hormonal changes.

Etiology:
- Abberation of Normal Development and Involution (ANDI)
- Exaggeration of normal proliferative and involutional changes
- Likely related to a predominance of estrogen over progesterone. Estrogen stimulates proliferation of fibrous and epithelial tissues.
- Most features affect the terminal duct lobular unit (TDLU)
  - Cystic dilation of the ductules of the lobule
  - Fibrosclerosis of the surrounding intralobular stroma
- There is increased production and increased absorption of fluid secreted by apocrine cells within the lobules

Key mechanisms / processes involved with FCC:
- Adenosis
  - Increase in the size and number of the ductules (acini) and lobules
  - Enlarged lobules/ TDLUs ~5-7 mm in diameter (normal lobular units typically measure 1- 2 mm)
- Epitheliosis – Epithelial hyperplasia
  - Increase in the number of epithelial cell layers within the ducts and lobules without an increase in the number of ducts or glands
- Stromal fibrosis
  - overgrowth of the fibrous connective tissues
- Duct ectasia; cyst formation; apocrine metaplasia
  - microcysts   (≤ 2 mm)
  - macrocysts (> 2 mm)
  - duct dilatation

Clinical features:
- Most clinically evident in women between ages 35-55 years
- Breast pain (mastodynia)
- Multiple breast lumps (typically indicating cysts)
- Pain and nodularity varies with menstrual cycle
- Nipple discharge from several ducts is occasionally present
- Symptoms typically regress after menopause

Sonographic features of FCC:
- Multiple cysts of varying sizes
- Microcyst cluster can appear as a thinly septated cyst (represent cystically dilated ductules within a lobule/ TDLU with intervening hyperechoic fibrous walls)
- Duct dilatation
- Increased echogenicity and attenuation of mammary layer (from stromal fibrosis)
- Enlarged lobules may occasionally be seen as small hypoechoic or isoechoic nodules; best seen when surrounded by hyperechoic fibrous stromal tissue

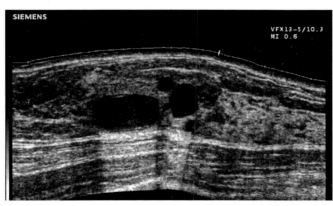

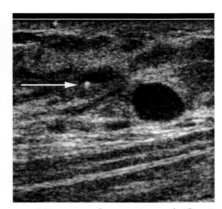

Fibrocystic change
(Courtesy: Siemens Medical)

Microcyst shows microcalcification

Calcifications related to FCC are better seen on a mammogram. On the sonogram, calcifications are occasionally seen with microcyst clusters and milk-of-calcium cysts, and with sclerosing adenosis (adenosis with reactive fibrosis).

FCC is a possible cause of nipple discharge. Discharge is usually bilateral and involves multiple duct orifices. Greenish or milky discharge that is only manually expressible is not considered suspicious. A bloody discharge is more uncommon and requires further evaluation.

Solid Nodules associated with FCC

Enlarged, isoechoic lobules or TDLUs measuring 5-7mm associated with adenosis may be difficult to differentiate from a true solid lesion. However, lobular enlargement related to FCC is usually bilateral and generally has a similar imaging pattern in each breast. Isolated or asymmetric nodules, especially in an older patient, are more worrisome for neoplastic change. When multiple enlarged TDLUs lie adjacent to each other, they can create a combined mass effect that can reach 2-3cm or more in size. This grouping of enlarged TDLUs has been termed "tumoral adenosis."

Sclerosing adenosis can appear as an enlarged isoechoic or hypoechoic TDLU, that may also have microlobulated margins and/or a central sclerotic echogenic focus. In some cases, sclerosing adenosis displays irregular or spiculated margins and shadowing, or appears as an area of architectural distortion, which can mimic cancer. Calcifications may be present but not always resolved.

A TDLU can be distended with solid material related to florid (papillary) duct hyperplasia or by papillary apocrine metaplasia.

Microcysts that are too small to resolve within an enlarging TDLU may appear echogenic, as opposed to cystic. Also some macrocysts can contain echogenic material from proteinaceous debris, foamy macrophages, white blood cells, red blood cells, which can give the TDLU or macrocyst a solid or a complex appearance.

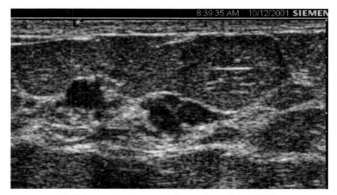

Solid-appearing nodules related to FCC.

B. Simple Breast Cyst

A breast cyst develops over time from progressive dilatation of the ductules within a lobule. Sonography's primary role is the differentiation of benign cysts from solid masses, which greatly impacts patient management.

Etiology:
- Feature of fibrocystic change
- Arise in terminal ductal lobular unit (TDLU)
- Obstruction of extralobular duct by epithelial proliferation or fibrosis
- Ductules / acini within lobule expand with fluid
- Retention of secretions leads to cyst formation
- Epithelial lining

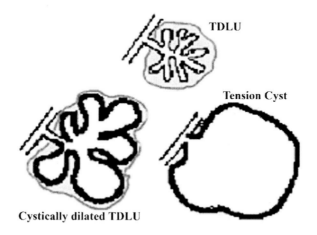

Clinical features of breast cysts:
- Most common single cause of a breast lump
- Occurrence more common between ages 35-50 years
- Single or multiple
- Mobile; compressible (unless tense)
- Cyclic tenderness; Size can vary with menstrual cycle
- Typically subside after menopause
- May persist after menopause in woman on HRT, digitalis (or medications that elevate estrogen levels)

Mammographic features:
- Round, oval shape
- Smooth, circumscribed margins
- Radiolucent halo sign (thin, lucent rim of compressed tissue around cyst – benign feature
- Water-density mass (can be low-high density relative to fat-density)

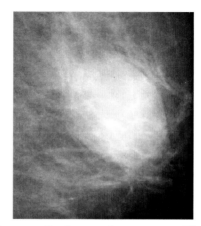

Mammogram of well-circumscribed water-density mass. The mass correlated with a cyst.

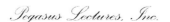

Sonographic features:
Diagnostic Criteria for Benign Simple Cyst
- Round, oval shape
- Smooth, thin-walls
- Anechoic
- Distal sound enhancement
- Thin, bilateral refractive edge shadowing

Additional features
- Compressibility with variable transducer pressure
  (round, "tense" cysts may show minimal compressibility)
- No internal vascular signal with Doppler

The walls of a simple cyst must be uniformly thin. Often the echogenic wall is nearly imperceptible.

The accuracy of a diagnosis of a benign simple cyst approaches 100% when all the diagnostic sonographic criteria are met.

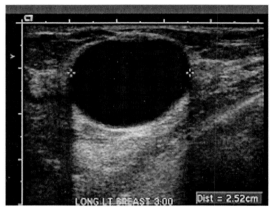

2.5 cm rounded tense simple cyst.

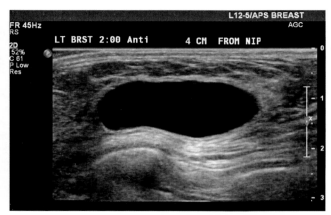

4 cm flaccid simple cyst.

Evaluation of Breast Cysts – Technical and Diagnostic Pitfalls
Sound enhancement is a useful artifact that is a diagnostic feature of a breast cyst. Demonstration of distal sound enhancement may be decreased if the cyst is:
- Small in size
- Surrounded by fibrous tissue
- Located deep in breast, adjacent to muscle
- Contains viscous material (see complex cyst section)
- Imaged with spatial compound imaging

Enhancement is often less evident when adjacent to hyperechoic, fibroglandular tissue. Spatial compounding can reduce the degree of enhancement beneath small cysts and eliminate edge shadowing.

Artifactual echoes within cyst can give a simple cyst a complex or solid appearance. Detrimental artifacts occur from:
- Excessive gain setting; noise, clutter, speckle
- Reverberation
- Poor focusing (volume averaging – slice thickness)
- Grating lobes; side lobes

Using higher frequency and focusing at the level of the cyst improves delineation the wall margins and internal contents, as well as enhancement effects. An acoustic offset may be needed to reduce slice thickness in the near field, especially when evaluating small, superficial cysts.

Before evaluating a cyst for benign or suspicious features, technical factors must be adjusted to eliminate detrimental artifacts. When altering technical parameters, care must be taken not to eliminate true echoes within a breast mass. Some solid masses can appear pseudocystic at low gain settings. It is important to optimize gain settings, dynamic range, frequency, and focus levels in order to resolve true echoes within a complicated cyst or markedly a hypoechoic solid mass.

C. Complicated – Complex Cysts

Breast cysts that display internal echoes or wall changes are termed complicated or complex cysts. The sonographic patterns of these masses do NOT meet the strict, diagnostic criteria of a benign simple cyst.

Newer high-resolution transducers are capable of detecting real particulate matter within cystic masses that generate echoes. In the majority of cases, these findings are benign, and related to fibrocystic changes. In much rarer cases, the internal echoes are a reflection of neoplastic change.

True echoes within a cystic breast mass can be related to:
- Protein globules
- Cellular debris
- Cholesterol crystals
- Foam cells; apocrine cells, epithelial cells
- Blood (red blood cells)
- Pus (white blood cells)
- Milky inspissated fluid
- Fibrous stroma
- Intracystic papillary tumor (rare)

Sonographic features include:
- Diffuse low-to-medium level internal echoes
- Fluid-debris levels
- Fat-fluid levels
- Thin or thick septations
- Concentric or eccentric wall thickening
- Mixed solid and cystic components

The degree of distal sound transmission can be diminished depending on the viscosity and contents of the mass.

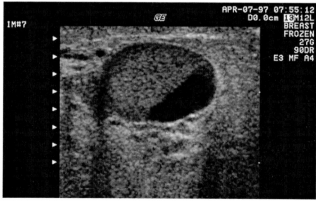

Fat-fluid level within cyst. The fat-laden fluid level is echogenic.

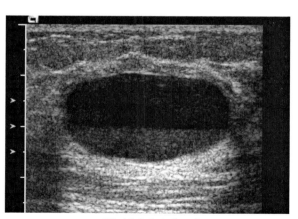

Fluid-debris level.

Methods that can induce movement of echoes within a breast cyst during sonographic evaluation include:
- Increasing the transmit power
- Insonating with color or power Doppler
- Applying dynamic transducer compression to shake particles
- Changing the patient's position

Lighter weight, subcellular particles are easily moved by increasing the sound energy (e.g., increasing output gain, applying Doppler). Heavier, non-attached particles may be moved with transducer pressure or positional changes.

Many complicated cysts with thin walls, and low-level internal echoes or fluid-debris levels, are usually related to benign fibrocystic changes.

Fat-fluid levels may take several minutes to shift when the patient is moved from a supine to an upright position. The echogenic fat layer will slowly move to the anterior, nondependent portion of the cyst. This feature helps to differentiate the echogenic fat layer from papillary apocrine metaplasia. Both entities can give the cyst an "acorn" like appearance. No blood flow will be detected within the echogenic material of either process.

Thin, internal septations usually represent the thin fibrous walls between cystically-dilated ductules within an enlarged TDLU, or cluster of simple cysts.

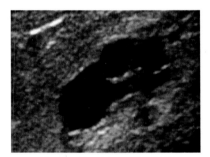

Cystically-dilated TDLU.

A milk-of-calcium cyst shows tiny, non-shadowing calcifications (calculi) along the dependent portion of the cyst. On the 90^0 lateral mammographic view with a horizontal x-ray beam, the calcium layer settles to the dependent portion of the cyst yielding a "teacup" appearance. This is a benign finding.

Sonographic findings worrisome for inflammation of a cyst include:
- Uniform, isoechoic wall thickening
- Possible fluid-debris levels
- Doppler detection of increased wall vascularity (hyperemia)

A fluid-debris layer associated with a thick, isoechoic wall suggests an acutely inflamed or infected cyst. Such cysts require aspiration with cytologic analysis, Gram stain, and culture and sensitivity.

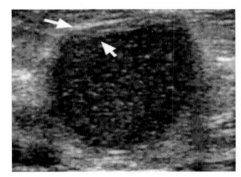

Thick, isoechoic wall thickening associated with cyst inflammation.

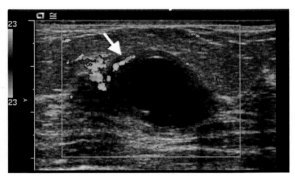

Color Doppler reveals hyperemia along thickened wall of this inflamed cyst.

Pegasus Lectures, Inc.

Sonographic features that are suspicious for possible neoplastic change within a cystic mass include:
- Thick isoechoic septations
- Certain mural nodules / eccentric wall thickening
- Doppler confirmation of a fibrovascular stalk
- Intracystic nodule with microlobulated, angular, ill-defined margins
- Loss of cyst wall definition or extension of tumor mass past cyst wall into the duct or into surrounding tissues

In most cases, mural nodules are related to benign proliferative disorders, such as papillary apocrine metaplasia, which is a feature of fibrocystic change. These changes occur within a thin-walled, pre-existing cyst.

Unlike papillary apocrine metaplasia, an intracystic papilloma or carcinoma is more likely to display microlobulated surfaces, a coarser and more echogenic internal echo pattern, and extension of the tumor past the cyst wall into the duct.

Doppler allows detection of blood flow within a fibrovascular stalk extending into an intracystic papillary lesion. Malignant intracystic nodules tend to show multiple feeding vessels into the tissue component of the mass. A benign intracystic papilloma tends to show only a single feeding vessel. Papillary apocrine metaplasia does not show blood flow within the intracystic echoes.

Sometimes a collection of pus, clotted blood, or sludge-like material can simulate a mural nodule. A nodule attached to the cyst wall will not move with changes in patient positioning or with compression techniques.

A solid neoplasm that has undergone cystic or hemorrhagic necrosis or degeneration can appear as a complex mass.

Aspiration and possible biopsy differentiates benign from malignant changes. A bloody aspirate is worrisome for malignancy. A purulent aspirate indicates infection.

Types of Complicated Cysts / Complex Cystic Breast Masses		
Foam cyst	Galactocele	Abscess
Acorn cyst	Sebaceous cyst	Hematoma
Fat-fluid level; PAM	Oil cyst –Fat Necrosis	Hemorrhagic cyst
Lipid cyst	Intracystic papilloma	Seroma
Infected cyst	Intracystic carcinoma	Papillary apocrine metaplasia
Apocrine metaplasia	Necrotic neoplasm	
	HNG-DCIS	

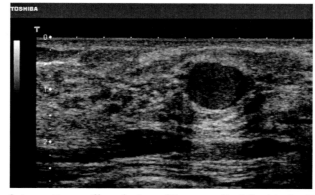

Intracystic papillary lesion. (Courtesy:Toshiba Medical)

D. Galactocele

A galatocele is a milk-filled retention cyst associated with lactation.

Etiology:
- Develops secondary to duct stasis and obstruction
- Milk-containing (inspissated fatty material)
- Typically occurs during or shortly after lactation
- Associated with abrupt cessation / suppression of lactation

Clinical features
- Palpable mass in pregnant or lactating woman
- Subareolar location most common
- Persistent galactocele can transform into an oil cyst
- Infected galactocele can lead to mastitis or abcess formation

Mammographic features:
- Well-circumscribed mass
- Variable density depending on fat content; often radiolucent
- Rim calcification possible

Sonographic features:
- Round, oval, or mildly lobulated
- Well-circumscribed, smooth margins
- Cystic mass with internal echoes generated from fatty contents
- Less often anechoic
- Distal sound enhancement, but may be less than with simple cyst
- Fat-fluid level possible
- Wall calcifcation associated with oil cyst
- Milky fluid upon aspiration is diagnostic of a galactocele.

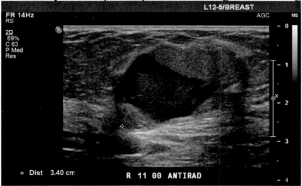 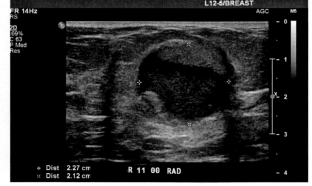

Galactocele with mixed echo pattern.   *A change in patient postion showed slow movement of echogenic internal echoes.*

E. Sebaceous Cyst - Epidermal Cyst

Sebaceous and epidermal cysts may be clinically indistinguishable.

Etiology:
- Small skin appendage mass
- Retention cyst resulting from obstructed sebaceous gland or hair follicle
- Contains sebum or keratin
- Epidermal inclusion cysts may also occur secondary to trauma.

Clinical features:
- Palpable, subcutaneous mass; can bulge skin
- Most common locations are near areola or at inferior breast
- May be associated with darkened skin pore
- May become inflamed and tender, especially if ruptured
- Ruptured, inflamed cyst can lead to abscess formation

Sonographic features:
- Subcutaneous location, typically involving the dermis
- May cause focal skin thickening
- Round or oval shape
- Well-circumscribed margins
- May be anechoic, or contain low-medium level internal echoes
- Posterior acoustic enhancement; variable degree

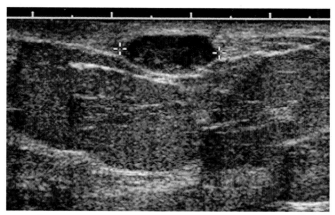

Sebaceous cyst involving the dermal layer of the skin.

The oily, waxy material within a sebaceous or epidermal cyst can cause low-to-medium level echoes. The excretory duct from the mass to the skin may occasionally be seen. Infected cysts may show increased wall thickening. Wall calcification may be seen with persistent masses.

Technical consideration:
Use of an acoustic stand-off pad or generous amounts of scanning gel help to optimize focusing at the superficial level of a sebaceous cyst.

Inflammatory Changes, Traumatic Changes & Radiation Effects

F. Puerperal (Lactational) Mastitis
Breast inflammation that occurs during lactation is called puerperal mastitis. This is the most common cause of "acute" mastitis.

Etiology:
- During lactation, bacteria can enter the breast through a crack in the nipple. This allows bacteria to enter a breast duct and occlude the duct orifice. The most common offending bacteria is Staphyloccus aureus. Milk stasis within the obstructed duct increases the risk of infection.
- Other pathways of infection include the bloodstream or ascension through the ducts.

Clinical features:
- Tender, edematous breast
- Skin thickening, reddening in region of plugged milk duct
- Possible purulent duct discharge
- Enlarged painful axillary nodes
- Leukocytosis and possible fever

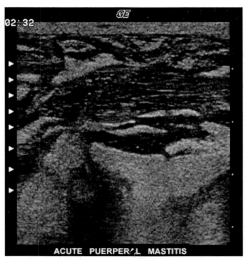

(Courtesy: GE Medical Systems)

Sonographic features of acute mastitis: (variable degree)
- Skin thickening with increased echogenicity
- Dilated lymph channels paralleling the skin
- Dilated ducts containing inspissated fluid
- Increase echogenicity of subcutaneous fat with poor delineation of fat /parenchymal interface
- Edematous parenchymal pattern; interstitial fluid
- Possible abscess formation

Doppler reveals hypervascularity of the affected tissues. Abscess is a complication of mastitis. Lactational mastitis usually resolves with antibiotic therapy. Clinical history helps to differentiate mastitis from inflammatory carcinoma.

G. Abscess

An abscess is a collection of purulent material (pus) within the breast associated with liquifactive tissue necrosis. Abscess formation is a complication of breast infection (mastitis). The pus-filled cavity can be unilocular or multilocular. Most breast abscesses are subareolar in location, but can be found at any level of the breast.

Predisposing factors:
- Puerperal mastitis
- Infected cyst (sebaceous, galactocele)
- Inverted nipple
- Mammary duct fistula
- Post-operative infection

Sonographic features of an abscess:
- Complex fluid mass with round, oval, or irregular shape
- Circumscribed, thick, or angular margins
- Anechoic, hypoechoic, and/or echogenic internal echoes
- May show septations
- Variable distal sound enhancement

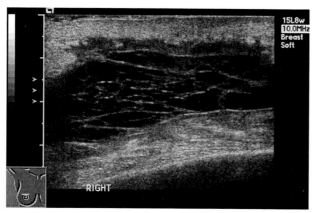

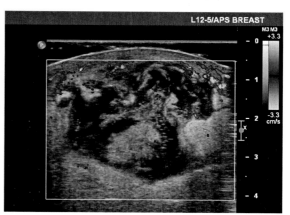

Breast abscess with septations and an increase in echogenicity of the adjacent, edematous tissues.

Color Doppler image shows hyperemia of adjacent edematous skin and tissues but no blood flow within the complex abscess cavity.

Doppler will show hyperemia along the walls of the abscess and in the surrounding tissues, but not within the fluid collection. Air within an abscess cavity can generate hyperechogenic foci.

An abscess may require drainage. Cytologic and bacteriologic analysis helps to differentiate bacterial from other causes of abscess formation, and to exclude malignant cells.

Inadequate treatment will lead to progressive tissue destruction. Residual effects of an abscess can include architectural distortion, fat necrosis, calcification, or focal scarring.

H. Duct Ectasia and Periductal Mastitis

Periductal mastitis is referred to as plasma cell mastitis, chronic mastitis, or as mammary duct ectasia, depending on the stage or histologic findings present. Periductal mastitis is a non-infectious form of mastitis and is of importance since certain clinical and imaging features can mimic carcinoma.

Unlike puerperal mastitis, periductal mastitis typically affects perimenopausal and postmenopausal women. Features are usually bilateral and involve subareolar structures. Overtime, the subareolar ducts become distended with thick, fatty, pasty secretions. Nipple discharge can be sticky, and green, milky, or bloody in coloration. Irritation of the nipple and areola from the discharged secretions can elicit symptoms that mimic Paget's disease. The secretions within the lactiferous ducts can cause chemical irritation and erosion of the duct wall. Leakage of secretions through an ulcerated duct can elicit an acute inflammatory reaction around the duct (periductal mastitis). The associated inflammation and periductal fibrosis can lead to nipple retraction. Duct fistula or rupture can lead to subareolar or periareolar abscess formation. Duct ectasia may also be associated with calcifications on a mammogram. The end-stage of the disease is fibrous obliteration of the duct lumen (mastitis obliterans).

Sonographic features of duct ectasia/periductal mastitis:
- Dilated subareolar ducts that contain anechoic fluid or diffuse echoes from inspissated material
- Possible duct wall thickening or ill-defined borders from periductal fibrosis (not always detectable)
- Doppler may show increased flow along duct wall
- Possible subareolar abscess
- Possible nipple retraction

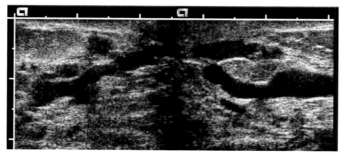

Subareolar ductal ectasia

I. Granulomatous Masititis

Granulomatous mastitis is a descriptive term and can be associated with a variety of conditions:

Foreign Bodies	Implants	Silicone
	Wax	Foam sponge
	Pacemaker	Catheters
	VP shunt	Mesh
	Sutures	Scar
	Metallic clip	Transsected hookwire
Specific Diseases	Tuberculosis	Actinomycosis
	Sarcoidosis	
Auto-Immune Disorders	Wegener granolomatosis	
	Giant cell arteritis	
	Polyarteritis	
Fungal Infection	Histoplasmosis	Blastomucosis
Parasitic Disease	Schistosomiasis	Hydatid disease
	Cysticerosis	Filariasis

Granuloma formation is a manifestation of inflammation. In the breast, foreign bodies, such as silicone, are common causes for granulomatous change. A granuloma produces a hard-firm breast mass.

J. Mondor's Disease

Mondor's disease represents thrombophlebitis of the superficial veins of the anterior chest and breast. In most cases, findings are unilateral. The etiology of this rare condition is often unknown. Predisposing factors include trauma, infection, recent surgery, cancer, or history of a hypercoagulable state.

Thrombosis causes an inflammatory response surrounding the vein. Recanalization of the vessel usually occurs over several months. The condition may recur.

Clinical features include:
• Sudden onset of breast or chest pain
• Development of a superficial cord-like mass
• Associated tenderness, erythema, and possible retraction of the overlying skin

Mammographic features:
• May show linear, nodular density
• May be normal

Sonographic features:
• Dilatation of the affected vein with internal echoes indicating clot
• Doppler shows absent/reduced blood flow in the clotted segment
• Adjacent skin may show focal thickening
• Adjacent tissues may show edematous changes

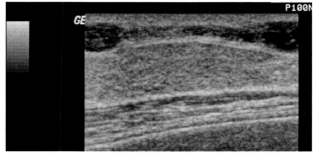

Thrombosed superficial breast vein.   *(Courtesy: Cindy Rapp)*

Pegasus Lectures, Inc.

Breast Trauma

Sonography is especially helpful to evaluate the patient with breast trauma. Mammography is often contraindicated in such patients.

Post-traumatic and post-surgical changes include:

Acute changes:
- Edema
- Skin thickening and bruising (contusion)
- Fluid collections (hematoma; seroma; or abscess from secondary infection)
- Fat necrosis (acute)

Late changes:
- Scar formation
- Skin and tissue retraction
- Fat necrosis (chronic)
- Oil cyst / lipophagic granuloma
- Dystrophic calcifications

K. Hematoma

A hematoma is a collection of blood within the breast related to vessel damage.

Etiology:
- Secondary to blunt trauma, surgery, aspiration, biopsy
- Increase risk in patient on anticoagulants
- Spontaneous hematoma associated with anticoagulants or bleeding disorders (thrombocytopenia, leukemia)

Clinical features:
- Skin bruising and thickening
- Breast tenderness; palpable mass

Sonographic features:
Features vary with the extent, duration, and degree of blood coagulation
- Complex fluid mass with variable distribution of internal echoes or septations (clotted blood is echogenic relative to fresh blood)
- Round, oval or irregular shape
- Wall thickening is common
- Variable amount of distal enhancement

Associated features:
- Overlying skin thickening
- Increased echogenicity of surrounding tissues from edema and tissue hemorrhage

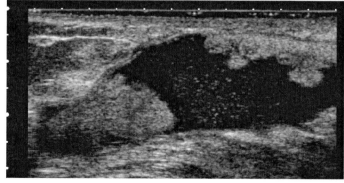

Post surgical hematoma with a complex appearance from liquid and clotted blood.

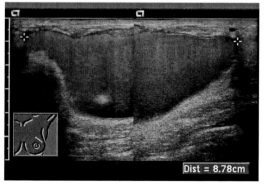

Hematoma secondary to traumatic seat belt injury with internal echoes generated from blood elements

Hematomas tend to become more sharply demarcated with age. Post-surgical hematomas can be irregular in shape. Bleeding from transected tissues can accumulate within the surgical cavity. Postoperative differential diagnosis of a complex appearing fluid collection includes seroma or abscess. Distinction of these entities is often based on clinical findings if the fluid collection is not drained.

A hematoma resolves over time but may cause residual effects that include Cooper's ligament thickening, architectural distortion, fat necrosis and/or scarring. These residual effects can mimic cancer.

L. Seroma
A seroma is a collection of serous fluid; or the watery portion of blood. A seroma that fills the surgical cavity after breast surgery helps to remold the breast's shape.

Clinical features:
- Palpable mass at surgical site (segmentectomy, ALND, mastectomy)
- May become large
- Formation of a seroma in the axilla following ALND can cause lymphedema of the arm and breast

Sonographic features:
- Shape conforms to surgical cavity; may be irregular
- Fluid-collection that may be anechoic or contain some low-level echoes
- May have septations
- Distal sound enhancement

Seromas are gradually absorbed by the body and do not need intervention unless large. Some persist for an extended period after surgery or reform.

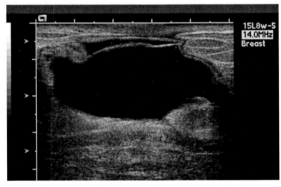

Seroma. (Courtesy: Siemens Medical)

M. Fat Necrosis
Localized trauma to the breast can cause focal hemorrhage and liquefaction of breast fat leading to necrosis and fibrosis. There are two distinct presentations of fat necrosis: a fibrotic mass that can mimic cancer, or as an oil cyst.

Etiology:
- Nonsuppurative inflammatory process
- Associated with trauma, surgery, irradiation, mastitis
- Feature of seat-belt injury; lumpectomy; reduction mammoplasty
- Can be idiopathic

Clinical features:
- Typically asymptomatic
- May present as firm-to-hard palpable mass; possible skin retraction
- More common in older women with large, fatty breasts
- Multiple oil cysts associated with nodular panniculitis
  (Weber-Christian disease)

Pegasus Lectures, Inc.

Mammographic features:
- Spiculated mass with possible central lucency
- Irregular mass with or without calcifications
- Oil-cyst: round or oval smooth-walled radiolucent mass with or without rim calcification
- Capsule sign: Thin, radiodense rim surrounding radiolucent fat-containing mass.

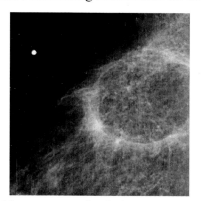

Mammogram of radiolucent oil cyst.

Sonographic features of fat necrosis (variable presentations):
- (Fibrotic form): Irregular or spiculated, ill-defined, hypoechoic mass with acoustic shadowing
- Complex mass
- (Oil cyst): Circumscribed, round or oval cystic mass; anechoic or low-medium level internal echoes; may show fat-fluid level; distal wall enhancement. Wall calcification causes hyperechoic walls and distal shadowing.

An oil-cyst will show thick, oily material upon aspiration.

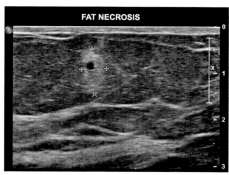

Fat necrosis seen as a hyperechoic region with central fluid in subcutaneous fat.

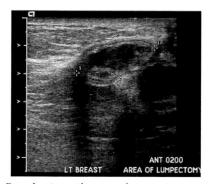

Developing oil cyst at lumpectomy site.

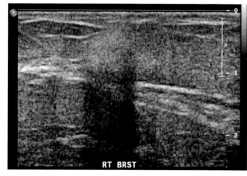

Fat necrosis with focal hyperechogenicity of the subcutaneous fat and distal shadowing.

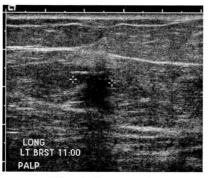

Fibrotic fat necrosis causing focal shadowing.

Patients that have undergone breast reduction surgery often show fat necrosis and scarring in the periareolar region and at the 6:00 incision site that extends from the nipple to the inframammary fold.

N. Scar

Scar formation is a late finding of breast trauma, surgery, and irradiation. Post-surgical scarring can affect the skin, subcutaneous tissues, and parenchymal tissues along the incision site. Over time, fluid-collections (seroma, hematoma, abscess) can be replaced by architectural distortion, fat, necrosis, and/or scarring. Any of these conditions can mimic cancer. Fat necrosis often accompanies scarring. The scar typically contracts and shrinks over time with fat accumulating in the center of the scar.

Etiology:
• Regenerative proliferation of connective tissue at injury site

Clinical features:
• Skin thickening, hardening, and possible retraction at incision site
• Possible firm, palpable mass beneath incision or at site of previous hematoma or abscess

Mammographic features:
• Increased radiodensity of affected tissues
• Elongated or spiculated mass effect usually associated with architectural distortion
• Changing appearance in different views
• May have associated calcification

Sonographic features:
• Skin thickening with possible retraction at scar site
• Irregular, ill-defined area of architectural distortion with posterior acoustic shadowing
• Appearance changes in orthogonal scan planes (key point)
• Degree of shadowing typically reduces with transducer pressure
• No vascularity with Doppler

The age of the scar affects its appearance. The effects of scarring typically diminish with time so serial examinations are helpful to differentiate a scar from local tumor recurrence.

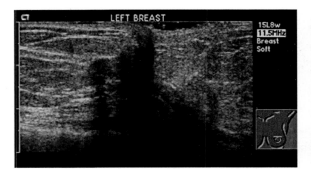 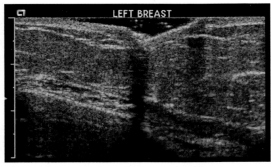

Post-operative scarring can have imaging patterns that mimic cancer. With scarring, the region of shadowing and interruption of tissue planes will vary in appearance in orthogonal scanning planes.

Technical considerations:
Using dynamic transducer compression is helpful when evaluating a scar. The shadowing appearance of the scar is in part due to refraction from the fibrotic tissues. In most cases, transducer compression will flatten the tissue fibers and decrease these effects (helping to differentiate a scar from cancer).

It is important to scan the full region of the scar in orthogonal planes. Following surgery, the spatial extent of the wound cavity and scar defect correlates with the path of the skin incision. Typically, the effects of the scar are wider and better seen in one plane. Scanning perpendicular to the scar often shows only a narrow region of discontinuity of the breast tissues.

Scar tissue does not elicit a Doppler signal, which may help differentiate a scar from a recurrent tumor.

Correlation of history with imaging features will avoid unnecessary biopsy.

Radiation Effects

Lumpectomy and radiation therapy are treatment options for stage 1 and stage 2 cancers. Post-operative changes are accentuated and prolonged in patients receiving radiation therapy. Effects diminish with time but some changes may take up to two years to resolve. Some skin thickening and tissue fibrosis or scarring may persist.

Post-irradiation changes can mimic or obscure malignancy.

Features and complications associated with lumpectomy and radiation therapy include:
- Skin edema, thickening and erythema (may show peau d'orage appearance)
- Parenchymal edema
- Vascular dilatation (radiotherapy induces hyperemia)
- Interstitial fluid or fluid-collections (seroma, hematoma)
- Dilated subdermal lymphatic channels
- Architectural distortion
- Fat necrosis
- Scar formation
- Calcifications

Edema causes breast swelling and increased tissue echogenicity. There is poorer differentiation between the subcutaneous fat, Cooper's ligaments, and parenchymal tissues. Scattering of the sound beam from edematous tissues reduce sound penetration of the breast. Edema also causes increased thickening and echogenicity of the skin.

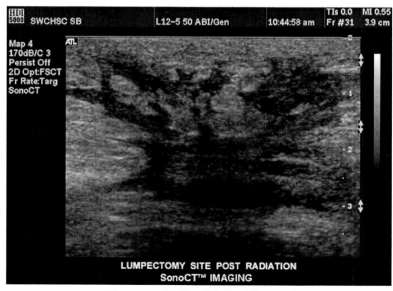

(Courtesy: Philips Medical Systems)

CHAPTER SEVEN

Breast Pathology
Benign Solid Masses

A. Fibroadenoma

Fibroadenoma is the most common benign solid breast tumor. This noninfiltrative lesion compresses surrounding tissues as it grows within normal tissue planes. The pseudocapsule of a fibroadenoma represents the leading edge of compressed breast tissue surrounding the mass.

Etiology – Histology:
- Estrogen-induced breast tumor
- Overgrowth of connective and glandular tissues within a lobule

Clinical features:
- Most common breast tumor in female under age 30; more common than cysts in this age group
- Develops in female of reproductive age; rarely after menopause
- Easily movable; firm, rubbery palpable mass
- Single or multiple; unilateral or bilateral
- Higher incidence of multiple, bilateral tumors in black women
- Tumors typically < 3 cm in size
- May grow rapidly during pregnancy
- Regress in size after menopause; may enlarge in woman on HRT

Older fibroadenomas can undergo hyalinization, degeneration, sclerosis, necrosis, and calcification.

Mammographic features include:
- Low-density to high-density (radiopaque) water-density mass
- Circumscribed, smooth margins
- Round, oval, or lobulated contour with distinctive notch
- Thin radiolucent halo-sign
- Occasional coarse popcorn-like or thin rim (eggshell) calcifications indicate degenerative changes

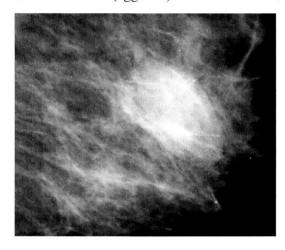

A fibroadenoma may be obscured and missed on a mammogram in the radiographic dense breast.

Sonographic features of fibroadenoma include:
- Wider-than-tall, ellipsoid shape; may show macrolobulation
- Oriented with long-axis parallel to skin
- Smooth, well-circumscribed margins – thin echogenic pseudocapsule
- Mildly hypoechoic or isoechoic when compared to fat
- Usually displays homogeneous echo pattern
- Normal sound transmission or mild sound enhancement
- Thin refractive edge shadowing is common

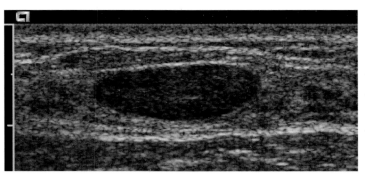

Fibroadenoma showing ellipsoid, wider-than-tall appearance.

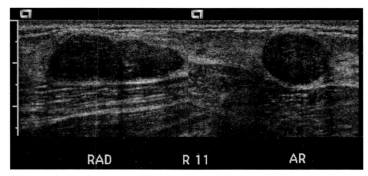

Fibroadenoma with gentle surface macrolobulations. This tumor is was not very compressible and indented the pectoralis muscle with transducer pressure.

On occasion, an internal fibrous septation may be seen as a thin, echogenic line that horizontally traverses the fibrodenoma. (This non-enhancing internal septa is a MRI feature of fibroadenoma.)

Fibroadenomas can be firm or mildly compressible with transducer pressure and will displace or indent adjacent structures. These features help to differentiate a fibroadenoma from a fat lobule. A fat lobule will be more compressible and will not indent fascial planes and muscles.

Fibroadenomas frequently show some peripheral and internal blood flow depending on tumor size and on Doppler sensitivity.

Fibroadenomas typically measure ≤ 3.0 cm in size, but can grow rapidly during pregnancy and lactation. Larger, rapidly growing masses should be differentiated from giant or juvenile fibroadenoma, lactating adenoma, phyllodes tumor, PASH, or medullary carcinoma.

Larger fibroadenomas are more likely to show more than 3 macrolobulations. Large tumors are more likely to be heterogeneous and show evidence of degeneration, sclerosis, or necrosis. Hyalinized fibroadenomas can display shadowing and some marginal irregularity.

After menopause, fibroadenomas tend to regress in size and/or calcify. Coarse popcorn-like calcifications on a mammogram are characteristics of a degenerating fibroadenoma. Thin egg-shell calcification occurs along the tumor rim. Calcified fibroadenomas display partial or complete acoustic shadowing and may mimic a suspicious lesion.

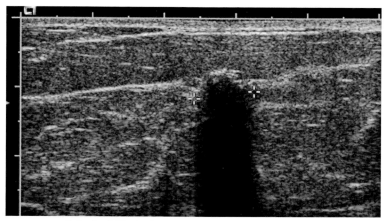

Calcified fibroadenoma with acoustic shadowing.

Variants of Fibroadenoma

1. **Complex Fibroadenoma**

    In some atypical cases, fibroadenomas can show internal epithelial proliferative changes that lie within the spectrum of fibrocystic change. Such changes can appear as small cystic areas, microcalcifications, or as a focal area of hyperechogenicity. These features may indicate internal apocrine metaplasia with cyst formation, epithelial calcifications, or sclerosing adenosis. Complex fibroadenomas are reported to show a slight increased relative risk for developing breast cancer.

    A rapidly growing fibroadenoma with internal cystic spaces should be biopsy to be differentiated from phyllodes tumor or medullary carcinoma.

2. **Juvenile Fibroadenoma**

    Juvenile fibroadenoma typically develops in an adolescent female before 20 years of age. Juvenile fibroadenoma accounts for 5-10% of fibroadenomas in this age group. This non-tender, well-circumscribed mass grows rapidly and is often large at time of presentation. Tumors often exceed 5cm in size and can distort the skin. Newer terminology for this giant type of fibroadenoma is *fibroadenoma with highly cellular stroma*. Tumors are often homogeneous and show distal sound enhancement. Doppler typically shows prominent vascularity.

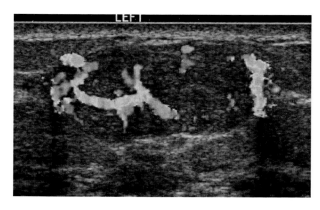

B. Lactating (Secretory) Adenoma

Lactating adenoma is a benign, well-circumscribed solid mass that grows rapidly during pregnancy and lactation in response to increased hormone stimulation. Surfaces can be microlobuated. The lesion primarily contains glandular elements. It is debated as to whether this tumor actually develops during pregnancy or reflects growth stimulation of a pre-existing fibroadenoma or tubular adenoma. Tumor regression follows cessation of lactation. Lactating adenomas can display increase echogencity and some internal small fluid areas related to secretory products.

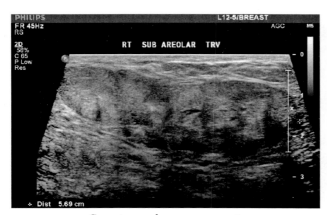

Secretory adenoma measuring 6 cm in lactating patient.

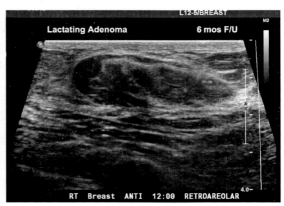

Follow-up exam in 6 months shows decrease in size following cessation of lactation.

C. Papilloma and Other Papillary Lesions

1. Intraductal (Large-Duct) Papilloma

A central papilloma grows within a major lactiferous duct beneath or near the areola (not in the TDLU). Current terminology for this lesion is large duct papilloma. Secretions from a papilloma can cause duct dilatation. Infarction and necrosis of the lesion can lead to intraductal bleeding. Intraductal papillary lesions slighty increase breast cancer risk.

Etiology – Histology:
- Frond-like proliferative mass within a major lactiferous duct
- Epithelial and myoepithelial cells cap the fibrovascular core

Clinical features:
- Incidence typically between ages 30-55 years
- Nipple discharge from a single duct
  Note: Intraductal papilloma is the most common cause of spontaneous bloody nipple discharge from a single duct.
- Palpable subareolar mass; may be nonpalpable   (Typically small but may grow to several centimeters)

Mammographic features:
Contrast ductography (galactography) allows detection of an intraductal mass. This procedure is discussed in Chapter 10.

Sonographic features include:
- Polypoid solid mass within fluid-distended main duct
- Circumscribed, solid subareolar or periareolar mass
- Typically isoechoic to fat, homogeneous, and nonshadowing
- Round, oval, or tubular shape
- Doppler flow confirms fibrovascular stalk

Pegasus Lectures, Inc.

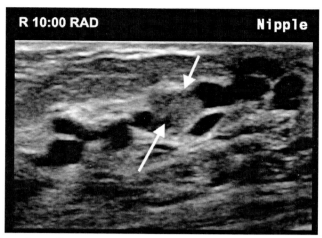

Intraductal papilloma seen as a solid mass within a dilated central duct.

Radial scanning best delineates the major subareolar ducts. A single dilated duct may indicate the presence of a tiny papilloma that is not apparent on standard imaging. Utilizing special maneuvers such as the rolled nipple technique, 2-handed peripheral compression, or upright scanning can better align the sound beam perpendicular to the subareolar duct.

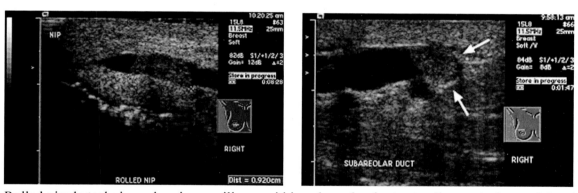

Rolled nipple technique showing papilloma within subareolar duct extending to the base of the nipple.

Large duct papillomas or papillary duct hyperplasias are the most common intraductal papillary lesions. However, some intraductal papillary lesions can undergo premalignant or malignant change. Although benign and malignant lesions can have similar sonographic appearances, papillary lesions that extend >1.5cm within the duct, expand the duct, or extend into branching ducts are more suspicious.

Ductography may be necessary to document the location and number of papillomas. Ultrasound can guide contrast injection into a distended duct if the nipple orifice is difficult to cannulate.

Some other entities that can produce intraductal echoes include inspissated secretions, clot, or fatty fluid within the duct. These materials will be movable when applying dynamic transducer pressure and will not show a fibrovascular stalk extending into the duct lumen with Doppler. Echogenic blood within a duct may obscure detection of a small papilloma. Doppler flow helps reveal the presence of an intraductal lesion and transducer compression will not fully collapse the duct around the mass. DCIS and papillary carcinoma care malignancies that produce intraductal lesions.

2. Intracystic Papilloma

Hypersecretion and blockage of a breast duct by an ingrowing papilloma can cause formation of a cyst around the soft-tissue mass. The cyst fluid can be bloody if there is torsion or infarction of the fibrovascular stalk. Unlike mammography, sonography can delineate both the solid and cystic components of the mass. The cyst walls must be carefully examined to delineate eccentric wall thickening or papillary tumor growth. Doppler flow within the solid component of a complex cyst differentiates mural tumor from a hemorrhagic cyst with clot or other cause of intracystic echoes.

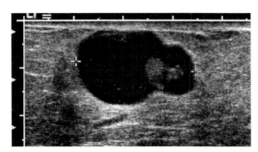
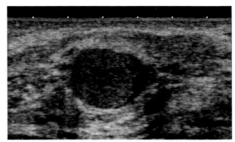

Intracystic papilloma
(Courtesy: Virginia Mason Medical Center, Seattle, WA)

(Courtesy: Toshiba Medical)

3. Multiple Peripheral Papillomatosis

Peripheral papillomatosis is characterized by multiple small, papillomatous growths that arise within a TDLU. Peripheral papillomatosis carries a higher risk for malignancy than a solitary, central, large duct papilloma.

4. Juvenile Papillomatosis

Juvenile papillomatosis typically affects adolescent and young women. Multiple small cysts interspersed with dense stroma give affected tissues a "Swiss-cheese" appearance, although some cases can simulate a solid mass. Associated breast changes include marked papillary hyperplasia, often with extreme atypia, which increases the future risk for breast cancer. Up to 28% of patients have positive family history of breast cancer.

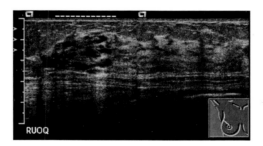

5. Nipple Adenoma

Nipple adenoma is an epithelial, papillary mass that grows within a duct that exits the nipple. This benign, circumscribed lesion can be a cause of nipple discharge and requires special sonographic technique (rolled nipple) to be imaged well.

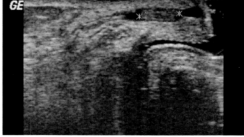

Rolled nipple technique displaying intraductal nipple mass.
(Courtesy: Cindy Rapp, BS, RDMS)

D. Lipoma

A true lipoma represents an overgrowth of adipose tissue encased by a thin connective tissue capsule. This compressible mass typically arises in the superficial fat layer of the breast. Echopalpation helps to correlate clinical with sonographic findings.

Clinical features:
- Movable, soft, compressible, superficial palpable mass
- May be large in size
- Small lipomas can be asymptomatic

Mammographic features:
- Radiolucent (fat-density) lesion
- Well-circumscribed with thin fibrous capsule
- Calcification is not a feature unless internal fat necrosis

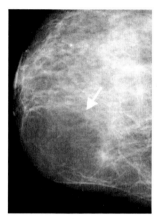

Mammogram of radiolucent lipoma.

Sonographic features:
- Round or oval shape
- Smooth, circumscribed, thinly encapsulated margins
- Isoechoic (to fat) or hyperechoic pattern
- Mild enhancement or normal sound transmission

Isoechoic lipomas may be difficult to differentiate from other fat lobules. Some isoechoic lipomas show numerous thin, internal echogenic septa. Lipomas are easily compressible with transducer pressure (~30%).

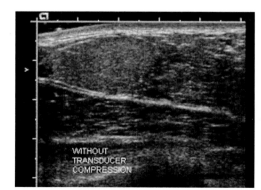
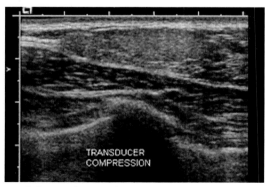

Palpable lipoma that shows compressibility with transducer pressure.

Some types of lipomas, including angiolipomas and fibrolipomas, tend to be uniformly hyperechoic. Another differential diagnosis is breast hemangioma.

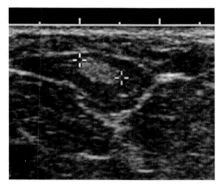

Hyperechoic subcutaneous lipomatous mass.

E. Hamartoma

Breast hamartomas are uncommon, intraglandular masses composed of varying amounts of normal or dyplastic breast tissues. These benign masses are also called fibroadenolipomas, lipofibroadenomas, and adenolipomas depending on the relative proportions of fibrous, glandular, and fatty tissues within the mass.

Etiology / Histology:
- Localized overgrowth of fibrous, epithelial, and adipose tissues
- Lacks true capsule; mass encased by a thin layer of connective tissue
- Epithelial – lobular elements may undergo fibrocystic changes

Clinical features:
- Often over 3cm in size
- Larger masses are palpable and movable
- Soft-to-firm; softness and compressibility depends on amount of fibrous tissue
- Most common locations are subareolar or in upper outer quadrant
- Can be associated with multiple hamartoma syndrome (Cowden's disease)

Mammographic features:
- Encapsulated island of mixed densities (fat and water densities) separated from normal ductal structures
- "Breast within a breast", sausage-like appearance
- Small lesions can be missed

Sonographic features:
- Oval or lobulated shape
- Smooth, thinly encapsulated mass with a heterogeneous echopattern (isoechoic fatty or lobular elements; hyperechoic fibrous elements; echogenic pseudocapsule)
- Some acoustic shadowing if high proportion of fibrous elements

The imaging pattern depends on the relative amounts of fat, glandular, and fibrous tissue present. Dynamic transducer pressure shows compressibility of a hamartoma, which is usually less compressible than a lipoma.

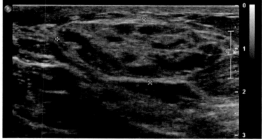

Breast Hamartoma

F. Focal Fibrosis

In some cases, the cause of a palpable or mammographic abnormality is benign focal fibrosis. Other names for this entity are fibrous mastopathy, chronic indutrative mastitis, and fibrous disease of the breast.

Etiology / Pathology:
- Focal accumulation of dense stromal fibrous tissue
- Does not contain mature lobules; paucity of ductal elements
- TDLU are atrophic, obliterated, or underdeveloped

Clinical features:
- More likely to develop in women during 4th – 5th decade of life
- More common in diabetic women
- Can present as palpable lump or be asymptomatic
- Most common site: Upper outer quadrant
- Not associated with a increased relative risk for breast cancer

Mammographic features:
- Nonspecific, asymmetric density or mass (Medium-to-high density)
- Suspicious calcifications uncommon

Sonographic features: (variable)
- Homogeneous intensely hyperechoic tissue (similar to dense interlobular fibrous tissue)
- Well-circumscribed but not encapsulated or ill-defined
- May cause architectural distortion and acoustic shadowing
- May appear as an isoechoic or hypoechoic nodule simulating a fibroadenoma

True focal fibrosis will be more uniformly hyperechoic than echogenic fibroglandular tissue that contains normal isoechoic ducts and lobules.

In the absence of any malignant features, pure hyperechogenicity is a benign sonographic feature.

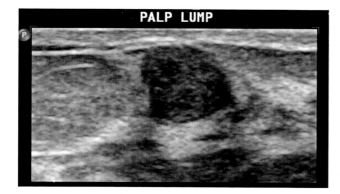
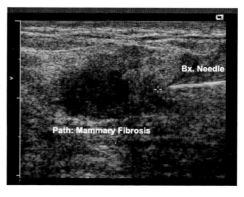
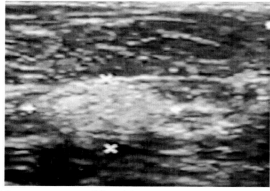
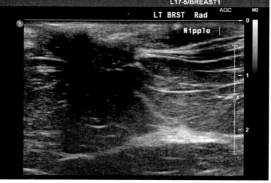

Variable appearance of focal fibrosis: Hypoechoic solid mass with circumscribed or ill-defined margins; hyperechoic mass (stromal fibrosis); architectural distortion with acoustic shadowing (simulating cancer).

G. Diabetic Mastopathy

Disorders in collagen metabolism are a feature of diabetes. Premenopausal, Type-I diabetic women are at increased risk of developing firm breast lumps related to benign fibrosis. These fibrous nodules can simulate cancer on clinical and imaging tests.

Clinical features:
- Firm, non-tender mass
- May be bilateral
- History of long duration Type 1 diabetes

Mammographic features:
- Nonspecific focal region of increased opacity
- May appear as irregular, spiculated mass
- May be missed in the radiographic dense breast

Sonographic features:
- Irregular, ill-defined, or spiculated mass
- Markedly hypoechoic; central hypoechoic focus
- May be taller-than-wide
- May show microlobuted surfaces
- Distal acoustic shadowing

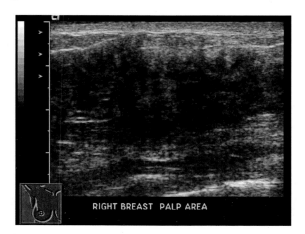

RIGHT BREAST PALP AREA

The imaging features of diabetic mastopathy can be similar to cancers with scirrhous features (low-intermediate grade IDC NOS, lobular or tubular carcinoma). Biopsy provides a definitive diagnosis.

Findings may be bilateral and muticentric.

No increased in Doppler flow is noted relative to adjacent tissues.

H. Other Benign Conditions

1. Pseudoangiomatous Stromal Hyperplasia

Pseudoangiomatous Stromal Hyperplasia (PASH) represents a focal overgrowth of stromal connective tissue that forms a breast mass. The stromal tissue contains avascular, lit-like cavities that look similar to vascular channels. This condition is thought to have a hormonal etiology related to a predominance of progesterone stimulation.

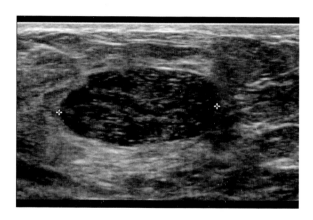

PASH: Rapidly growing circumscribed solid oval mass containing small cystic spaces that mimics fibroadenoma.

Clinically palpable masses are firm, mobile, and nontender. PASH tends to develop in premenopausal women or in postmenopausal women taking combination estrogen-progesterone hormone replacement therapy.

On imaging tests, PASH can mimic fibroadenoma. Sonographically, a PASH nodule appears as an ellipsoid, well-circumscribed, solid mass. In some cases, PASH nodules contain areas of fibrocystic change. Internal cysts yield an imaging pattern similar to that of a complex fibroadenoma or possibly phyllodes tumors.

PASH can grow and recur if not fully excised.

2. Radial Scar

A radial scar (sclerosing duct hyperplasia) is not related to previous trauma or surgery. Use of this term should not be confused with post-surgical scarring, although both conditions can show similar imaging features. Lesions > 1cm in size are called complex sclerosing lesions. The etiology is unclear. Tumors are comprised of spicules of proliferating epithelium that radiate out from a central fibrous core.

On a mammogram, a radial scar often appears as a spiculated lesion with a small, radiolucent, fatty center (black star pattern). On a sonogram, this ill-defined mass shows acoustic shadowing or localized architectural distortion. Imaging features mimic carcinoma.

Although a radial scar is classified as benign, it has been theorized to be a precursor to tubular carcinoma, and can be associated with atypia.

3. Granular Cell Tumor

Granular cell tumor (GCT) is though to arise from Schwann's cells of the peripheral nerves. Originally, the mass was thought to originate from muscle tissues and was termed myoblastoma. A GCT rarely develops in the breast, although lesions can occur in many other parts of the body. Both men and women can be affected. Occurrence is more common between ages 30-50 years. Tumors most often reside in the upper outer breast quadrant and typically measure less than 3cm.

Although benign, GCT is important because it can simulate invasive breast carcinoma on clinical and imaging examinations. Palpable tumors can be firm, fixed, and may show associated skin dimpling. Histologic analysis is necessary to differentiate this mass from cancer, and to avoid unnecessary radical surgery. Typically, local excision with wide margins is curative.

On a sonogram, a GCT can appear as an irregular or spiculated mass with a hypoechoic central nidus and distal shadowing. A change in transducer angle may alter the apparent echogenicity of the mass. The lesion displays a high fibrous component.

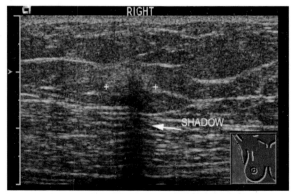

Small granular cell tumor showing echogenic halo, subtle spiculation, hypoechoic central nidus and shadowing.

• CHAPTER EIGHT •

Malignant Breast Pathology
Specific Malignant Masses, Metastases and Tumor Recurrence

A. General Breast Cancer Facts
- Breast cancer is the most common malignancy in American women, excluding skin cancer.
- For a woman living to age 85, the odds of developing breast cancer is estimated to be 1 in 8 women (~ 13%). Incidence is highest in postmenopausal women.
- Breast cancer is the second leading cause of cancer death in American women. (Lung cancer is the leading cause.)
- Only about 20% of breast lumps are cancerous; 80% are benign.
- Most breast cancers develop in women with no family history of the disease. (< 16-25% breast cancer is genetically linked.)
- In women, most breast cancers develop in the upper outer quadrant where there is the greatest amount of glandular tissue.
- Cancers progressively enlarge, independent of the menstrual cycle.
- Early detection of cancer improves survival rates.
- Cancers larger than 1 cm in size have an increased risk of nodal involvement.
- Tumor size, multicentricity, lymph node involvement, and distant metastases are major prognostic indicators and affect surgical planning and breast conservation options.

Risk factors for breast cancer in females include:
- advancing age
- personal or family history of breast cancer
- benign proliferative disease with atypia
- early menarche; late menopause
- late age for first pregnancy
- nulliparity
- high-dose radiation exposure
- exogenous estrogen use
- post menopausal obesity

More than 80% of breast cancers occur in women older than 50 years of age. In the USA, caucasian women are more likely to develop breast cancer, however, African American women have the highest mortality rates.

B. Major Histologic Types of Breast Cancer
Major classifications of breast cancer are listed below:

1. Invasive Carcinomas   (~80% of all breast malignancies)
- Invasive ductal carcinoma, not otherwise specified (NOS)
  (60-70% of all breast cancers; ~80-85% of all invasive carcinomas)
- Invasive lobular carcinoma   (~10%)
- Special-type invasive duct carcinomas
  - Tubular   (~ 2-8%)
  - Medullary   (~ 5%)
  - Colloid   (~ 2%)
  - Papillary   (~ 2%)

2. **Non-invasive Carcinomas (~20% of all breast malignacies)**
   - Ductal carcinoma in situ (DCIS) = intraductal carcinoma (85% of non-invasive cancers)
   - Lobular carcinoma in situ (LCIS) = lobular neoplasia

   (The reported incidence of DCIS is now much higher due to mammographic screening.)

Most breast cancers arise in breast ducts or lobules.

Ductal carcinomas tend to arise within the extralobular terminal duct (ELTD) of the terminal duct lobular unit (TDLU), at or near its junction with the lobule. Malignant cells can then extend down the ELTD into the main duct, and also extend into the smaller ducts of the lobule.

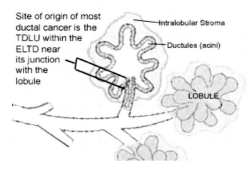

Non-invasive (in-situ) carcinoma is localized to the site of origin. Malignant epithelial cells are confined to the duct and do not extend past the basement membrane. Since cancer cells have not gained access to the blood vessels or lymphatic channels, there is essentially no risk of metastasis.

Invasive (infiltrating) carcinoma spread past the site of origin. Tumor cells grow past the basement membrane of the duct wall into the surrounding tissues. Such cancers can gain access to lymphatic channels and blood vessels lying near the duct. Tumor cells can then travel to the lymph nodes and distant sites, potentially causing metastases. Invasive tumors increase morbidity and mortality.

Breast malignancy is divided into four major histological categories:
- Tumors of ductal epithelial origin (adenocarcinoma)
- Tumors of lobular origin
- Tumors of stromal tissue
- Metastatic disease to the breast

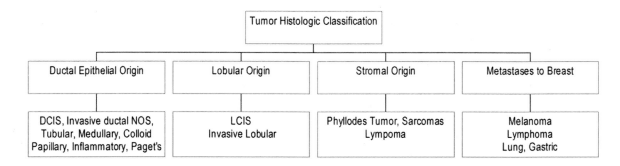

Breast malignancies display significant differences in morphology and histology. The imaging features of a cancer varies greatly depending on its composition, its growth rate, and the on the body's response to the presence of the tumor. Morphologically, cancers can range in appearance from spiculated-to-circumscribed, and often display a combination of features.

102

C. Ductal Carcinoma in Situ (DCIS)

Ductal carcinoma in situ (DCIS) is the most common noninvasive breast malignancy. Another name for this cancer is intraductal carcinoma. DCIS is the earliest identifiable form of breast cancer. In past years, DCIS only represented about 10% of malignancies. Since the widespread use of screening mammography, breast cancer is now being detected much earlier state. As a result, DCIS now accounts for 20-40% of detected malignancies.

Etiology:
- Malignant transformation of epithelial cells lining the duct without extension past the duct wall into the surrounding tissues
- Typically arises in ELTD of TDLU near its junction with the lobule

Clinical features:
- Usually asymptomatic; diagnosed by screening mammography
- Occasionally, a palpable mass of variable size, shape, and consistency
- Possible nipple discharge (serous, bloody)

Main types of DCIS by grade:
- Low nuclear grade / "non-comedo type"
  This is a well-differentiated from of DCIS and includes cribiform, micropapillary, and solid types. Atypical ductal hyperplasia is a precursor lesion. Lesions are comprised of smaller, more uniform cells, and have a better prognosis than higher-grade lesions. Mammography can underestimate the size of noncomedo DCIS since some of these cancers do not show calcification, or display lower density peripheral microcalcifications.
- Intermediate grade
- High nuclear grade / "comedo type"
  This is a poorly-differentiated, more aggressive form of DCIS. This cancer progresses to invasive carcinoma more quickly, and recurs faster, than other in situ lesions. Large neoplastic cells fill the duct. Characteristic features include duct distension with plug-like, necrotic (cheese-like) material that contains extensive calcifications. The distended ducts often shows periductal fibrosis and inflammation.

Mammographic features:
- Microcalcifications = earliest mammographic sign of breast cancer
  (~ 90% comedo DCIS cases; ~ 50% noncomedo cases)
  (Calcifications are often heterogeneous, vary in shape and size, and follow the duct line.)
- Features other than calcifications: (less common)
  - Nodular mass with / without calcifications
  - Non-specific soft-tissue density; asymmetric density
  - Solitary or multiple dilated ducts
  - Architectural distortion – can indicate invasive component

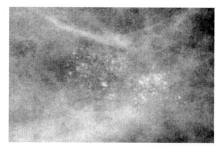 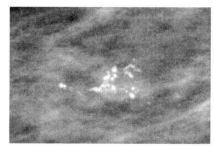

Fainter calcifications / Noncomedo DCIS   *Dense calcifications / Comedo DCIS*
(Courtesy: Fischer Imaging)

Generally, mammography is more effective at diagnosing DCIS than sonography since microcalcifications are often the primary feature. Mammographic sensitivity for DCIS is 70-80% with calcifications being the most common diagnostic clue.

Sonographic features of DCIS:
- No findings may be seen if tumor cells do not grossly distend the duct
- Distended duct with internal echoes with/without microcalcifications
- Tubular appearing soft-tissue intraductal mass
- Microlobulated solid mass with duct extension, branch pattern
- Intracystic papillary lesion

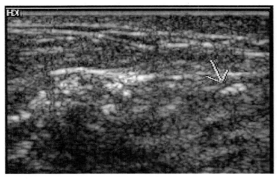

High nuclear grade DCIS with duct calcifications
Courtesy: Cindy Rapp, BS, RDMS

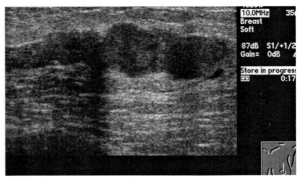

DCIS seen as tubular mass, solid intraductal mass
GSRMC, Corvallis, OR

Sonography has limitations regarding the diagnosis of DCIS. Malignant cells may be present without grossly distending the duct or TDLU. Microcalcifications are often difficult to resolve. There are also benign entities can cause duct distension, wall thickening, and/or intraluminal echoes. These include intraductal papilloma, papillomatosis, hyperplasia and other benign proliferative disorders, as well as, and periductal mastitis.

Other forms of DCIS

1. **Intracystic Papillary Carcinoma**
   Most papillary carcinomas are non-invasive. A papillary carcinoma growing within a duct can obstruct the duct and cause formation of a cyst. The cystic component of the mass may become palpable. Blood may fill the cyst cavity if there is infarction or torsion of the fibrovascular stalk. Nipple discharge may be present.

   Sonography is especially useful at showing mural tumor within this complex cystic mass. Extension of tumor past the cyst wall and margin irregularity or microlobulation increases the suspicion of malignancy, but these features may be seen with an intracystic papilloma.

2. **Paget's Disease of the Nipple**
   Paget's disease is an uncommon presentation of breast cancer that involves the epidermal layer of the nipple and is usually associated with underlying DCIS. Malignant cells spread along a subareolar duct and extend to the nipple and areola.

   Clinical features include erythema, ulceration, and eczema-like crusting of the nipple, as well as nipple discharge and itching. Progression to invasive carcinoma affects survival rates.

   Paget disease can be diagnosed clinically, without the need of sonography. Mammography may show subareolar microcalcifications. Sonography may be helpful to evaluate a coexistent subareolar mass.

D. Lobular Carcinoma in Situ (LCIS)

Lobular carcinoma in situ (LCIS) is not considered a true cancer and is referred to as lobular neoplasia. The significance of LCIS is that of being a marker for increased risk of the future development of invasive ductal or lobular carcinoma in either breast.

Etiology:
- Arises in the epithelium of the blunt ductules (acini) within the lobule
- Does not breach the basement membrane
- Typically multicentric (70%) and bilateral (30%)

Clinical features:
- Tends to affect premenopausal women; especially 44-54 years of age
- No palpable mass or specific physical finding

Mammographic and Sonographic features:
- Typically not detect by mammography or by sonography because of the absence of microcalcifications or formation of a discrete mass
- Rarely presents as a mass with/without calcifications
  (The dense breast tissue in younger patients can obscure findings on a mammogram.)

LCIS is typically diagnosed microscopically as an incidental finding from a breast biopsy performed for other reasons.

E. Invasive Ductal Carcinoma

Invasive ductal carcinoma, not otherwise specified (IDC NOS), is the most common breast cancer accounting for approximately 80% of all invasive breast malignancies. This type of breast cancer has no specific histologic features for subclassification as a "special-type" of breast cancer. Overall, IDC NOS has the worst prognosis of all breast cancers.

The body's typical response to an invasive carcinoma is to wall off the tumor with fibrous tissue to limit invasion. This fibroelastic host response is termed desmoplasia or reactive fibrosis. Cancers that produce significant desmoplasia are termed scirrhous-type lesions. Most IDC NOS tumors display scirrhous features. With slower growing tumors, the body has more time to incite a fibrous response. On gross specimen, scirrhous lesions are hard and gritty with irregular or stellate (spiculated) margins. Often these lesions contain a paucity of tumor cells, with a large part of the mass effect being composed of fibrous tissue.

Less often, IDC NOS tumors are highly cellular, circumscribed, and relatively soft. These tumors can grow fast and may show central necrosis.

Etiology - Histology:
- Malignant epithelial cells grow past the duct wall and invade surrounding fat / connective tissues
- Stroma typically contains a large amount of collagen

Clinically suspicious features:
- Firm, fixed, usually painless palpable mass
- Palpable size often larger than mammographic size
- Possible nipple discharge (most suspicious if bloody)
- Skin or nipple retraction

Mammographic features: (spectrum of findings)
- Asymmetric, high-density, spiculated or irregular mass
- Suspicious pattern of microcalcifications
- Architectural distortion
- Less often: circumscribed mass

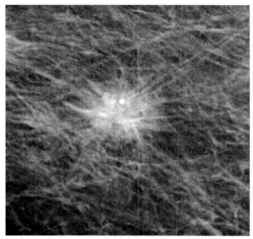

Mammogram of IDC with spiculated margins.

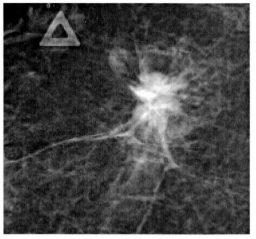

Invasive ductal carcinoma.

Associated findings
- Thickened, straightened, retracted Cooper's ligaments
- Duct dilatation; nipple retraction; skin thickening or dimpling

Sonographic features: (The more features displayed; the higher the suspicion of malignancy.)
- Spiculation (and/or thick echogenic halo)
- Angular margins
- Microlobulation
- Taller-than-wide
- Marked hypoechogenicity
- Microcalcification
- Acoustic shadowing
- Duct extension (intraductal component)
- Branch pattern (intraductal components)

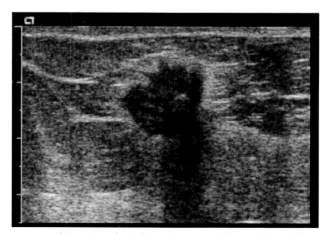

Sonogram of invasive ductal carcinoma with suspicious features.

A "classic" IDC NOS tumor presents as a spiculated mass on a mammogram. Since such lesions receive a BI-RADS 5 classification, they are often referred for biopsy rather than adjunctive sonographic imaging. Masses referred for ultrasound evaluation may show a variety of ultrasound features depending on tumor morphology, growth pattern, and the body's response to the presence of the mass. As mentioned before, IDC NOS can range in appearance from spiculated-to-circumscribed, or show a combination of findings. Some slow-growing, lower grade tumors contain fewer tumor cells and are mainly composed of reactive fibrous tissue, where as, fast growing, higher grade lesions are often highly cellular.

On a sonogram, IDC-NOS usually displays irregular, angular margins or spiculation that causes indistinct borders. A common appearance is a tumor with a thick echognic halo, hypoechoic central nidus, and distal shadowing. The thick, ill-defined, echogenic halo can represent tiny spicules within the infiltrative margin of the mass. High-resolution transducers can better resolve these tiny spicules especially along the lateral sides of the mass (due to perpendicular insonation). Long spicules radiating out from an infiltrative tumor may resemble retracted Cooper's ligaments.

IDC NOS often causes partial or complete acoustic shadowing. The degree of shadowing is usually related to the amount of fibrous tissue within or around the mass. Slow growing tumors have more time to elicit a fibrous response. Shadowing is more common with low-to-intermediate grade IDC tumors. Transducer compression will not eliminate malignant shadowing.

The orientation of IDC NOS tumors can be directed perpendicular to the skin. Small tumors growing within a vertically-oriented TDLU are more likely to be taller-than-wide. IDC NOS tumors are also more likely to grow across tissue planes.

In about one-third of cases, IDC NOS tumors have relatively circumscribed margins. Although this presentation is more characteristic of medullary, colloid, and papillary cancers, IDC NOS is the most common histologic type of breast cancer to present as a circumscribed or partially circumscribed mass. Often, these are highly cellular, higher-grade lesions. Rapid growth of the tumor does not allow the body enough time to elicit a fibrous response. Instead, fast growing cancers tend to elicit an inflammatory response (peritumoral edema) that can also cause an increase in tissue echogenicity adjacent to the mass. Highly cellular tumors are usually markedly hypoechoic and often display surface microlobulation. Tumors ≥ 1.5cm in size typically exhibit distal sound enhancement. Large tumors can show central necrosis. Hypercellular tumors often display prominent vascularity with Doppler. Hypocellular, fibrotic tumors tend to elicit less Doppler flow.

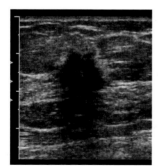 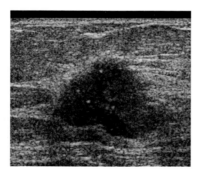 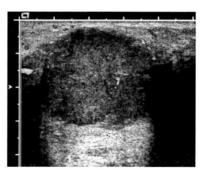

Low-grade IDC NOS with acoustic shadowing. *Intermediate grade IDC with combination of circumscribed and spiculated margins.* *High-grade IDC with relatively well-circumscribed margins and distal sound enhancement.*

Scanning in radial and antiradial planes allows better detection of intraductal components of tumor such as duct extension and branch pattern.

Secondary features are common with invasive cancers. Reactive fibrosis can cause thickening, straightening, and retraction of Cooper's ligaments. This can lead to skin dimpling or nipple retraction. Disruption of tissue planes occurs with invasion. An increase in the echogenicity of the subcutaneous fat accompanies tumor extension into the premammary layer. Interruption of the fat/dermal interface signifies skin invasion and is accompanied by focal skin thickening. Tumor extension through the retromammary fat and deep fascia will cause focal fixation of the breast to the muscle layer.

Architectural distortion without a mass is a less common presentation of IDC-NOS.

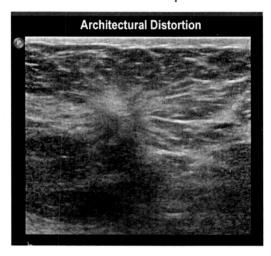

Architectural Distortion

Suspicious lesions are classified as BI-RADS® categories 4 or 5. Pre-operative or surgical biopsy is indicated for a definitive diagnosis.

Benign masses or conditions that display imaging features that mimic invasive carcinoma include:
- fat necrosis
- radial scar
- sclerosing adenosis
- scar
- fibrosclerosis
- fibrous (diabetic) mastopathy
- granular cell tumor

These benign masses can show ill-defined, irregular or spiculated margins and acoustic shadowing. Acoustic shadowing can be caused by a hyalinized or calcified fibroadenoma. Critical angle shadowing from Cooper's ligament can mimic malignant shadowing but is easily eliminated with transducer pressure.

F. **Invasive Lobular Carcinoma**
   Invasive lobular carcinoma (ILC) is the second most common invasive breast malignancy. This cancer is often multicentric and bilateral. ILC is the most frequently missed invasive breast cancer by physical examination or by mammography. Although ILC often has a diffusely infiltrative growth pattern, it may not produce specific clinical findings. When the disease is clinically evident, the cancer is often advanced. Breast density can limit mammographic detection of ILC in younger women. Since detection may be delayed until the disease is advanced, the prognosis can be worse for ILC than for other forms of breast carcinoma. In 30-50% of cases, patients will develop a second primary in the same or opposite breast within 20 years. A high percentage of women with ILC have coexistent LCIS.

   Etiology – Histology:
   - Small tumor cells infiltrate the surrounding stroma in single file rows (Indian file pattern)
   - Circumferential infiltration can occur around ducts and lobules (Targetoid pattern)

Clinical features: (variable presentation)
- May be asymptomatic
- Non-specific area of asymmetric thickening or induration
- Ill-defined, firm mass
- Multiple, small hard areas of nodularity
- Mean age at diagnosis: 45-56 years
  (Compared to other types of invasive cancers, ILC is least likely to present as a discrete palpable mass.)

Mammographic features: (variable presentation)
(Mammography can miss or underestimate ILC since suspicious calcifications are uncommon and the pattern of invasion can be diffuse and nonspecific.)
- Asymmetric parenchymal density, with / without architectural distortion
- Spiculated, ill-defined mass (less common)
- Retraction of glandular tissue and Cooper's ligaments
- Only ~ 10% have associated microcalcifications
- No findings are possible

Sonographic features of ILC:
(Findings can vary depending on whether ILC is diffusely infiltrative or forms a focal mass.)
- Ill-defined areas of hypoechogenicity within more hyperechoic fibrous stromal tissue that often cause shadowing (diffuse, infiltrative pattern)
- Hypoechoic mass with poorly-marginated, spiculated or angular margins, and distal acoustic shadowing (similar to IDC NOS)
- Architectural distortion

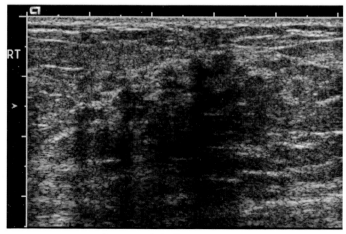

Invasive lobular carcinoma

Although findings can be nonspecific, sonography is often better at detecting alterations in breast tissues associated with ILC than mammography, especially in younger patients with radiographic dense breasts. Diffuse, infiltrative ILC can be difficult to differentiate from proliferative changes related to FCC and benign causes of shadowing. Vocal fremitus may help to differentiate normal from abnormal tissues.

The shadowing seen with ILC is typically not related to desmoplasia. Instead, it is likely caused by alteration in the axes of normal fibrous stromal tissue infiltrated by rows of ILC tumor cells. ILC tends to grow into the surrounding tissue like "roots" in single columns of cells, as opposed to forming a focal, expansile mass. Dynamic transducer pressure should be applied to distinguish Cooper's ligament shadowing from malignant shadowing.

As with mammography, ILC can be missed by sonography. MRI can be more helpful at assessing the extent of ILC prior to treatment.

G. Tubular Carcinoma

Tubular carcinoma is an uncommon, well-differentiated form of invasive ductal carcinoma. There are pure and mixed variants. Pure tumors are typically small (often < 1cm) and slow growing. Tumors of this type have an excellent prognosis and a very low incidence of axillary metastases. Tubular carcinoma is strongly associated with LCIS and a positive family history of breast cancer. Tumor foci can be bilateral and multicentric.

Unlike other "special" subtypes of invasive duct carcinomas, tubular carcinoma typically displays spiculated margins. Histologically, tubular carcinoma can be confused with sclerosing adenosis and radial scars.

Like low-grade IDC NOS, tubular carcinomas are hard, gritty, stellate lesions that incite marked desmoplasia (reactive fibrosis). Since tumors are typically small, tubular carcinomas may be detected on a screening mammogram before becoming clinically palpable.

Clinical features:
- Small, fixed palpable mass
- Skin dimpling may occur

Mammographic features:
- Small spiculated, radiodense mass
- Calcifications are common
- Satellite lesions; multicentric disease

Sonographic features:
- Small ill-defined or spiculated mass, may show angular margins
- Thick echogenic halo; hypoechoic central nidus; posterior shadowing
- Small lesions may be taller-than-wide
- Possible Cooper's ligament retraction; skin dimpling

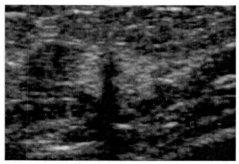

Small tubular carcinoma

H. Medullary Carcinoma

Medullary carcinoma is a "special" histologic subtype of invasive duct carcinoma, and accounts for ≤ 5% of all breast malignancies. This highly cellular cancer tends to develop earlier than most other breast cancers, and represents 11% of breast cancers in women under age 35 years. Characteristically, a medullary carcinoma is well-circumscribed with an expansile growth pattern. Tumors grow rapidly, can become large, and can undergo central necrosis. Tumors do not incite significant reactive fibrosis.

Pure medullary cancers have a moderately low incidence of lymph node involvement, and are usually associated with a good prognosis. Atypical tumors have more infiltrative features and a poorer prognosis.

Histologic features:
- Highly cellular tumor with high-grade, cytologic atypia
- Moderate-severe infiltration by lymphocytes or plasma cells within tumor and at periphery
- Central hemorrhage and necrosis (larger lesions)

Clinical features:
- Often smooth; round or lobulated
- Mobile, non-tender, and mildly compressible
- Rapid growth
- Often 2-3cm in size; large tumors can distort the breast
- Often located near the periphery of the breast

Mammographic features: (can simulate fibroadenoma)
- Round or lobulated, radiodense, circumscribed mass
- Pushing border may show radiolucent halo-sign
- Lacks microcalcifications
- Atypical tumors show more ill-distinct margins

Sonographic features:
- Round or oval shape
- Smoothly circumscribed or partially circumscribed margins
- Often show multilobulated or microlobulated surfaces
- May be taller-than-wide
- Hypoechoic-to-markedly hypoechoic internal echoes
- May show central cystic degeneration
- Typically shows distal sound enhancement

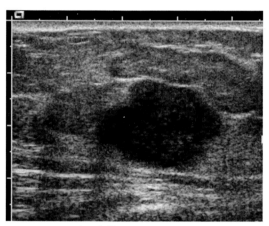

Medullary carcinoma

Dynamic transducer compression may show tumor compressibility. Close inspection of the tumor margins may show some surface lobulation or microlobulation, which raise the suspicion of malignancy. Larger tumors tend to undergo internal hemorrhage or necrosis, causing textural heterogenicity or cystic spaces. Tumors can be markedly hypoechoic or appear pseudocystic at lower gain setting. Internal Doppler vascularity confirms solid nature of mass.

On occasion, a thick, echogenic rim is seen around a rapidly growing medullary carcinoma that is related to peritumoral edema. A fast growing carcinoma can elicit an inflammatory response rather than a desmoplastic response to the presence of the tumor.

I. Colloid (Mucinous) Carcinoma

Colloid (mucinous) carcinoma is another "special" subtype of duct carcinoma. Unlike medullary tumors, colloid carcinoma usually grows slowly, rarely undergoes central necrosis, and is more likely to occur in older women. There are pure and mixed variants of this uncommon cancer that affect imaging appearance and prognosis.

A pure tumor is typically a well-circumscribed, lobulated mass that is relatively soft and gelatinous. These tumors have a low rate of axillary metastases and a good prognosis. Mixed variants contain less mucin, are often larger, and more infiltrative than pure tumors.

Histologic features:
- Cluster of uniform cells floating in large pools of extracellular mucin
- Small, uniform tumor cells with mild or moderate cytologic atypia

Clinical features:
- Smooth or lobulated palpable mass
- Mildly compressible and movable
- Represent a high percentage of cancers that develop in women over the age of 75 years

Mammographic features:
- Smooth, round or lobulated; low-radiodense mass
- May show some trabecular distortion
- Calcifications uncommon unless associated with DCIS

Sonographic features include:
- Smooth, circumscribed margins; thin echogenic capsule
- Can show microlobulated surfaces
- Isoechoic or hypoechoic as compared to fat
- Homogeneous to mildly heterogeneous texture
- Larger tumors often show distal enhancement

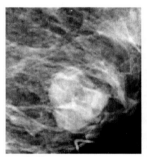
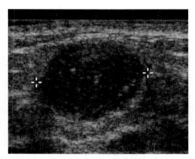
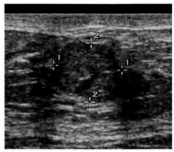

Colloid carcinoma: Mammogram of well-circumscribed water-density mass.

Colloid carcinoma: Sonogram of well-circumscribed hypoechoic mass.

Colloid carcinoma that is nearly isoechoic to fat with sound enhancement.

Close inspection of a colloid carcinoma will often display at least one or more suspicious characteristics such as: hypoechogenicity, microlobulation, possible duct extension or branch pattern. Small tumors can be taller-than-wide. Central necrosis is uncommon. Mixed tumors may show more surface and textural inhomogenicity.

Isoechoic tumors can mimic a lipoma, fat lobule, or even fibroadenoma. Smaller tumors are more likely to be isoechoic to fat.

Acoustic shadowing is not a feature of colloid carcinoma since these tumors do not cause reactive fibrosis.

J. Papillary Carcinoma

Invasive papillary carcinoma is rare and occurs most often in older women. Papillary carcinoma has a slower growth rate and a better prognosis than IDC NOS. Most papillary carcinomas are noninvasive lesions. Even invasive papillary carcinomas are relatively well-circumscribed tumors that may show only focal areas of invasion.

Etiology - Histology:
- (Central lesion) Frond-like epithelial tumor within large duct; lacks myoepithelial cells; can arise within pre-existing papilloma
- (Peripheral lesion) Arises within TDLU from areas of florid duct hyperplasia / papillomatosis
- Stromal or vascular invasion differentiates in situ from invasive lesions; Tumors cells tend to have low nuclear grade

112

Clinical features:
- Bloody nipple discharge is the earliest sign (from infarction or torsion of papillae)
- Subareolar palpable mass (central lesion)
- Larger mass may bulge the overlying skin
- Possible skin dimpling, ulceration, nipple retraction

Mammographic features:
- Solitary, central, circumscribed mass; may show focally obscured or ill-defined margins
- Cluster of circumscribed nodules in one breast quadrant
- Microcalcifications possible

Sonographic features:
- Relatively well-circumscribed solid mass (better seen if outlined by fluid within a dilated duct)
- Tend to expand duct and can involve branching ducts
- Small lesion may be taller-than-wide
- Can show surface microlobulation, irregularity, duct extension; branch pattern
- Microcalcifications occasionally resolved
- Doppler blood flow within fibrovascular stalk

Intracystic papillary carcinoma
- Intracystic mural nodule with duct extension past cyst wall
- Solid nodular component may show microlobulation or irregular shape
- Complex cyst with thick isoechoic septations
- Doppler flow within solid component

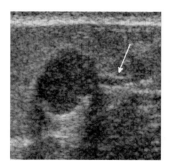 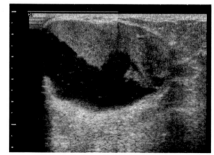 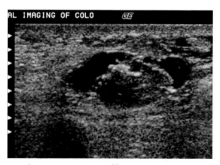

Papillary carcinoma *Invasive intracystic carcinoma* *Intracystic papillary carcinoma*
(Courtesy: Cindy Rapp, BS, RDMS)

Imaging features of invasive papillary carcinoma is often indistinguishable from in-situ or benign papillary lesions. However, the presence of any suspicious feature (microlobulation, angular margins, microcalcifications, intraductal components) will prompt a BI-RADS 4 classification and biopsy will allow a definite diagnosis. Compared to a benign large duct papilloma, malignant intraductal papillary lesions are more likely to extend >1.5cm within the duct, expand the duct, or extend into branching ducts.

Invasive intracystic papillary carcinomas appear as complex lesions. Doppler helps to differentiate an intracystic papillary neoplasm from inspissated material, clot, fat-fluid levels, or papillary apocrine metaplasia. Nonpapillary intracystic carcinomas can occur when a cancer secondarily invades the wall of an adjacent cyst or when a rapidly growing cancer undergoes extensive cystic necrosis.

Peripherally located invasive papillary carcinomas may appear as an enlarged, distorted TDLU.

Reactive fibrosis is uncommon with papillary carcinoma so shadowing is not typically seen.

K. Phyllodes Tumor

Phyllodes tumor is an uncommon fibroepithelial mass that is usually benign but can undergo malignant transformation and potentially metastasize. This tumor is the most common breast sarcoma, and previously known as cystosarcoma phylloides. Recurrence is possible if excision is incomplete.

A phyllodes tumor is considered the malignant counterpart of fibroadenoma. Larger tumors are more likely to be malignant. Hematogenous metastases occur mainly to the lung, pleura, bone, liver. Lymph node metastasis is rare.

Phyllodes tumors develop more often in women between the ages of 45-50 years, which is later than that typical for fibroadenoma.

Etiology – Histology:
* Fibroepithelial tumor with leaf-like (phyllodes) growth pattern
* Contains cyst-like clefts of mucus, hemorrhagic, or cystic fluid
* Stromal component can undergo malignant transformation in ~ 25 % of cases

Clinical features:
* Rapidly enlarging, nontender, firm, moveable palpable mass
* Large mass may bulge, stretch, discolor, and ulcerate the skin
* Dilated veins visible beneath overlying skin
* Solitary, unilateral
* Often smoothly lobulated

Mammographic features:
* Generally well-circumscribed, noncalcified, radiopaque mass
* May be focally invasive with ill-defined margin
* Dilated veins with larger lesions

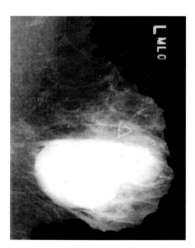

Sonographic features:
* Round, oval, lobulated, or polylobulated
* Usually circumscribed; but malignant mass may show focally ill-defined or irregular margination
* Hypoechoic solid mass with/without detectable internal cystic cavities
* Normal or enhanced distal transmission
* Doppler often shows prominent tumor vascularity.

Malignant lesions are more likely to grow rapidly, become polylobulated, and show focal areas of margin irregularity.

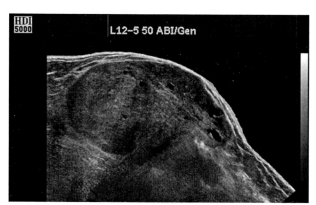

Large phyllodes tumor displaying internal cystic cavities.
(Courtesy: Philips Medical Systems)
(Reprinted with permission from SDMS/Pegasus Breast Ultrasound Exam Simulation CD, 2003)

L. Lymphoma

Lymphoma rarely presents as a primary breast cancer ($\leq 0.5\%$ of breast malignancies). Most lymphomas are secondary lesions, so knowledge of the patient's medical history is vital. Lymphoma can present as a nodular mass or as an indistinct, diffuse infiltrative process. Focal tumors are highly cellular. In many cases, lymphoma presents as abnormally enlarged intramammary or axillary lymph nodes. The most common lymphoma affecting the breast is Non-Hodgkin's lymphoma.

Clinical features:
- Palpable, rapidly growing breast mass(es)
- Possible skin retraction, erythema, and thickening
- Enlarged axillary lymph nodes

Mammographic features:
Nodular Pattern
- Single or multiple; round, oval, or lobulated
- Well-circumscribed or ill-defined
Diffuse Pattern
- Diffuse pattern with increased parenchymal density
- Skin thickening

Sonographic features include:
- Round or oval mass(es)
- More often circumscribed than ill-defined margins
- Tumors usually markedly hypoechoic; generally homogeneous
- Usually distal sound enhancement
- Possible skin thickening; dilated subdermal lymphatics

Markedly hypoechoic tumors may mimic a cystic mass. Doppler, however, will show internal vascularity within the lymphomatous lesion. Peritumoral inflammation and edema may cause hyperechogenicity around the tumor.

A diffuse pattern may simulate inflammatory carcinoma.

Biopsy is needed to differentiate hematologic malignancies, such as lymphomas or leukemias, from other nodular masses, or from inflammatory carcinoma.

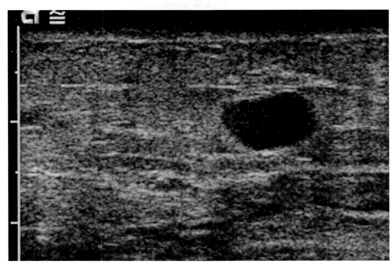
Well-circumscribed, markedly hypoechoic lymphoma.

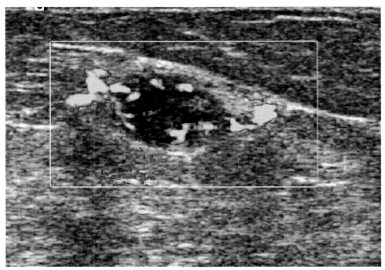
Marked flow within lymphomatous mass.
(Courtesy: B.Fornage MD)

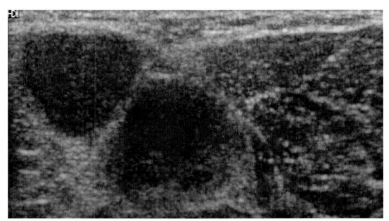
Enlarged, rounded, marked hypoechoic axillary nodes, with absence of fatty hila.
(Courtesy: Cindy Rapp, BS, RDMS)

M. Multifocal – Multicentric Carcinoma

Multifocality
A multifocal cancer refers to the presence of additional tumors within one breast quadrant or within the same ductal system as the primary tumor.

Multicentricity
Multicentricity refers to the presence of multiple tumors in different quadrants of the breast, or tumors separated by a distance of ≥ 5cm. Multicentric tumors are less common and may be of the same or different histologic types.

Breast malignancies that are multifocal or multicentric are more likely to recur, and typically have a poorer prognosis. Within the breast, cancer cells can travel from the primary lesion via the ducts to form satellite lesions. IDC NOS is multifocal in 25-50% of cases.

The presence of multiple or bilateral lesions alters surgical options and usually requires more extensive surgery for treatment purposes. Failure to remove all the tumor foci and intraductal components can compromise treatment outcome.

Whole breast sonography is helpful for assessing the presence of additional tumor foci in a woman with a known breast cancer. The addition of radial and antiradial scanning in the region of the mass will better allow detection of intraductal tumor that can lead to satellite lesions. Satellite lesion can be obscured on a mammogram in the patient with radiographic dense breasts.

Contrast-enhanced MRI plays is effective in the evaluation of multifocal, multicentric, and bilateral disease, as well as lymph node assessment in cancer patients.

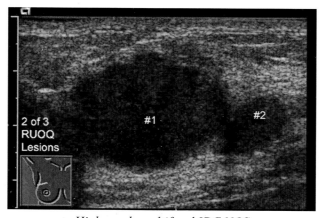

High-grade multifocal IDC NOS

N. Inflammatory Carcinoma
Inflammatory (diffuse) carcinoma is rare and accounts for about 1% of all breast cancers. This carcinoma is not a histologic subtype, but describes breast changes that occur when tumor cells from a highly aggressive cancer invade and block the lymphatic channels of the skin. Since malignant spread is rapid and diffuse, the prognosis is typically poor.

Tumor emboli within the dermal lymphatics cause characteristic, edematous skin changes. In the pure form, a primary lesion may not be evident. In other cases, a primary tumor, multifocal or multicentric lesions may be detected. Although this condition is usually unilateral, tumor cells can spread through lymphatic channels crossing the mid chest, and involve the opposite breast.

Histologic types:
- High-grade invasive ductal carcinoma (most common)
- Can be of other histologic types and grades

Clinical features:
- Skin erythema, edema and thickening causing "orange-peel" (peau d'orange) appearance that affects more than one-third of the breast
- Skin warmth; dilated veins
- Flat or retracted nipple
- Swollen, tender, hard breast
- Palpable mass not always present
- Enlarged axillary lymph nodes

Mammographic features:
- Affected breast is denser, larger, and less compressible
- Diffuse skin and trabecular thickening
- Hazy, increased density from tissue edema
- Dominant mass may be absent or obscured by increased breast density
- Lymphadenopathy

Sonographic features:
(Features include signs of inflammation in addition to suspicious changes)
- Diffuse skin thickening with increased echogenicity
- Dilated superficial veins
- Dilated subdermal lymphatic channels or presence of interstitial fluid
- Increased echogenicity of the subcutaneous fat
- Obscured/disrupted fascial planes
- Parenchyma may show diffuse, heterogeneous pattern with irregular shadowing
- Focal suspicious mass(es) may/may not be seen
- Thickened, echogenic Cooper's ligaments

Doppler often shows hypervascularity of tissues.

Axillary adenopathy is common. An extended sonographic examination can help show additional areas of adenopathy not seen on the mammogram (parasternal, infraclavicular, supraclavicular).

The clinical features of inflammatory carcinoma can mimic mastitis.

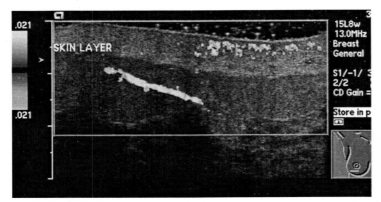

Inflammatory carcinoma showing marked thickening and increased echogenicity of the skin. Doppler shows hypervascularity.

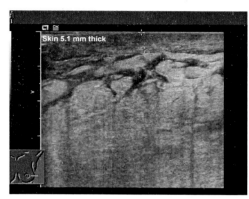

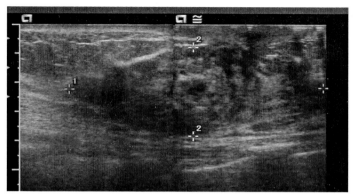

Skin thickening, dilated subdermal lymphatic channels, and parenchyal edema.

Inflammatory carcinoma: Large high grade invasive ductal carcinoma extending to skin in patient.

O. Cancer Staging

Stage 0	In situ (DCIS)
Stage 1	Small tumor < 2 cm No axillary lymph node involvement (negative nodes) No distant metastasis
Stage 2	Tumor ≤ 2 cm; Positive axillary lymph nodes; No distant metastasis (or) Tumor 2-5 cm; Positive axillary lymph nodes; No distant metastasis (or) Tumor > 5cm; Negative axillary lymph nodes; No distant metastasis
Stage 3	Tumor > 5cm in size Extensive local and regional spread (or) Tumor fixed to pectoralis muscle (or) Tumor with axillary lymph nodes fixed together in a matted axillary mass
Stage 4	Nodal involvement Distant metastasis present Tumor of any size with direct extension to skin or chest wall

Tumor size (T), the involvement of regional lymph nodes (N), and the presence or absence of distant metastasis (M) are components of the TNM Classification System.

Stage 1 tumors show well-differentiated cells, while stage 4 tumors are very poorly differentiated.

Tumor staging affects patient management and prognosis. Women with stage 1 or 2 breast cancer are offer breast conserving surgery, followed by radiation. Some cases require more extensive surgery. Adjuvant systemic therapy may include chemotherapy and/or hormonal therapy (e.g., tamoxifen). Higher stage cancers require more extensive surgery (including radical mastectomy), systemic therapy, and possibly radiation treatments.

P. Metastatic Disease

Cancer can spread from or to the breast by the following routes:
- Lymphatic channels
- Bloodstream
- Direct extension

1. Metastases from the Breast to Regional Lymph Nodes

Regional lymph node involvement is an important prognostic indicator of breast cancer. Axillary lymph nodes are the most common site of nodal metastases since most lymph from the breast (75%) drains to these nodes.

For purposes of cancer staging and prognosis, the level of lymph node involvement is important. Regional lymph nodes include:
- Level I, II, III axillary lymph nodes (Rotter's nodes are included with level II nodes)
- Ipsilateral internal mammary nodes
- (Supraclavicular lymph nodes)*
  (Important note: Until recently, positive supraclavicular lymph nodes were classified as "distant" metastases (M1) since metastasis occurs in a retrograde fashion at the confluence of the jugular and subclavian veins. Positive supraclavicular nodes are a late finding, but have recently been reclassified as "regional" lymph node involvement (N3) using the revised TNM staging system.)

When level III (subclavicular) nodes are positive, tumor cells have gained access to the bloodstream. Sonography or MRI can help identify lymph nodes that are too high or too deep to be clinically palpated or seen on a mammogram. Sonographically, internal mammary (parasternal) nodes are usually only seen when enlarged by metastasis.

Sonographic features suggesting nodal metastasis include:
- Nodal enlargement
- Round or lobular shape
- Asymmetric cortical thickening
- Irregular or ill-defined margins
- Marked hypoechogenicity or heterogeneous pattern
- Displaced, compressed, or absent hilar fat

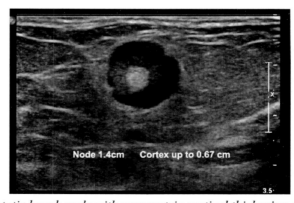

Round, markedly hypoechoic metastatic lymph node with asymmetric cortical thickening and compressed fatty hilum.

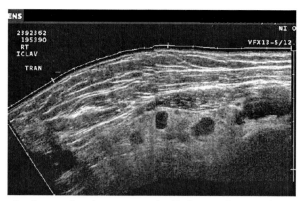

Infraclavicular lymphadenopathy showing markedly hypoechoic nodes with loss of fatty hila.
(Courtesy: B.Fornage MD, MD Anderson Medical Center, Texas)

It is not always possible to differentiate metastatic nodes from normal or reactive nodes. However, marked ipsilateral involvement on the side of the breast with suspicious findings suggests metastatic change rather than inflammation. However, mastitis or local infection may also show regional nodal changes. Metastatic nodes are more likely to show increased vascularity with multiple feeding vessels that extend through the capsule and cortex. Enlarged, reactive or inflamed lymph nodes tend to show a uniformly thickened cortex. Although inflammation can cause an increase in blood flow, a single hilar artery usually feeds the inflamed node.

Sonography can help assess regional lymph nodes in patients with known or suspected breast cancer. Patients with larger tumors, extensive intraductal components of tumor (duct extension, branch pattern), or show mutifocal or multicentric lesions are at more risk for nodal involvement. Besides the axillary nodes, sonography can sometime detects enlarged nodes in the supraclavicular and internal mammary regions. Internal mammary (parasternal) nodes are more likely to be involved when there is a medially located cancer. However, even lateral cancers can divert lymph to the parasternal chain, especially when the axillary lymph channels become obstructed.

2. **Hematogenous Metastases to Distant Sites**
    Metastases can spread from the breast to a distant site via the bloodstream. The most common sites of hematogenous metastases include:
    *   Bone (most common distant site)
    *   Lung
    *   Brain
    *   Liver

3. **Metastasic Disease to the Breast**
    Metastatic lesions within the breast are rare (1-5% of malignancies) and can arise from:
    *   A contralateral breast cancer (most common)
    *   Extramammary primary
    *   Hematological malignancies

    a. Metastasis from the Contralateral Breast
        Breast cancer cells can travel to the contralateral breast via lymphatic channels that cross the anterior chest, and via the blood.

        Contralateral breast metastasis often causes diffuse architectural distortion of the tissues without a focal mass. Diffuse skin thickening is often present. This pattern can mimic inflammatory carcinoma.

b. Metastasis from an Extramammary Primary Cancer
Metastasis to the breast from an extramammary primary cancer is rare. Tumor cells primarily reach the breast via the bloodstream. Some non-mammary sources include:
- Melanoma (most common in females)
- Lung
- Ovary
- Sarcoma
- GI tract

In males, prostate cancer is the most common primary to metastasize to the breast.

Metastatic tumors from extramammary sites are often solitary, but can be multiple and bilateral. Tumors are usually nodular in appearance and are fast growing. Metastases are often deposited in the subcutaneous fat layer near the skin. These metastatic tumors are usually circumscribed and show minimal, if any, fibrotic host response. Palpable masses are more likely to be smooth, rounded, and somewhat movable. There is usually no skin dimpling or retraction. The palpable size correlates well with mammographic findings.

Sonographic features of a metastatic breast lesion typically include:
- May show superficial location, often in upper outer quadrant
- Round, oval, or lobulated shape
- Hypoechoic solid mass(es), often with circumscribed margins
- Homogeneous to mildly heterogeneous echotexture
- Normal or mildly enhanced distal sound transmission

Often metastases (especially melanoma) show prominent vascularity with Doppler. Although these masses can simulate benign lesions, a metastasis should be considered in the differential diagnosis of a new breast mass in a patient with a history of a non-breast primary cancer.

(Ovarian metastasis may display a more diffuse infiltrative pattern.)

c. Metastasis to the breast from a hematologic malignancy
Lymphoma and leukemia are the most common lymphoreticular and hematopoietic malignancies to metastasize to the breast. Non-Hodgkin's lymphoma is the most common.

Sonographic features of metastatic lymphoma:
Focal nodular or diffuse pattern
- Focal lesions are markedly hypoechoic, homogeneous, with distal sound enhancement.
- Diffuse involvement shows hypoechoic glandular thickening.
- Multiple enlarged lymph nodes are present.

Q. Tumor Recurrence
Recurrent tumor can be difficult to distinguish from scar or fat necrosis. Recurrent carcinomas often have an unusual growth pattern and may spread diffusely, as opposed to forming a discrete mass.

Approach to determining tumor recurrence:
- Serial mammography with clinical examination to monitor changes
- Adjunctive sonography, especially in a woman with dense breasts (Although shadowing from scarring can obscure recurrent tumor)
- Supplemental contrast-enhanced MRI can help differentiate an older scar from recurrent tumor

Often tumor recurrence does not appear until 2 or more years following conservative therapy.

Mammographic features suggesting tumor recurrence at the lumpectomy site include:
- New, nodular, or ill-defined mass in area of previously stable findings
- Enlarging scar
- Increasing architectural distortion
- Associated suspicious microcalcifications
- Diffuse increased density

Sonographic features include:
- New hypoechoic, nodular or ill-defined mass; may show shadowing
- Maintains relative shape in orthogonal scan planes
- Presence of associated Doppler flow increases suspicion
- Mass or shadowing does not change significantly with transducer compression
- Enlarging area of architectural change

• CHAPTER NINE •

The Male Breast
Anatomy, Gynecomastia and Cancer

A. Normal Breast Anatomy

The normal adult male breast primarily consists of fat and connective tissue, as well as some rudimentary subareolar ducts. There is little secondary ductal branching. Since the male breast does not function to produce milk, lobules rarely form. The skin layer is thicker, and the pectoralis muscle is larger, in a male than in a female.

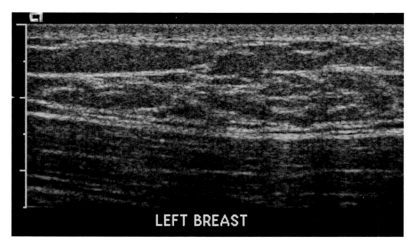

Sonogram of normal male breast demonstrating skin, fatty and connective tissues.

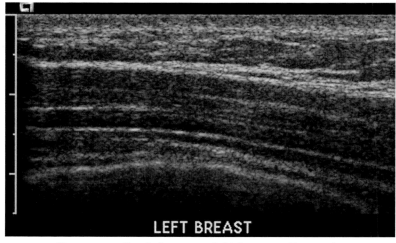

Sonogram of male breast and thick pectoralis muscle.

B. Male Breast Examination and Breast Disease

Symptoms leading to male breast examination include breast enlargement, tenderness, palpable lump, and/or nipple discharge. Mammography of the male breast is usually possible, although technically difficult to perform on the small breast size. High-resolution sonography is effective at detecting male breast pathology, characterizing mammographic abnormalities, and for guiding needle-biopsy of suspicious lesions and lymph nodes.

Many of the pathologies found in the female breast can occur in the male breast, although occurrence is less common. The most frequent benign disorder, gynecomastia, involves ductal and periductal connective tissues. Stimulated ductal tissue can also elicit intraductal and intracystic papillary lesions. Other benign masses include lipoma (most common focal mass), abscess, hematoma, and sebaceous cyst. Fibrocystic changes, fibroadenoma, and adenosis rarely occur since lobules do not fully develop in males.

Men do not undergo routine mammographic screening since the incidence of male breast cancer is so rare. Male breast cancer can be primary, secondary, affect the lymph nodes and spread to distant sites.

C. Gynecomastia

Gynecomastia represents non-neoplastic male breast enlargement and is the most common male breast disorder. The name for this condition comes from the Greek language and means, "woman-like breasts."

Gynecomastia results from proliferation of the subareolar ducts and the surrounding periductal stroma, as well as an increased deposition of subcutaneous fat. Estrogenic stimulation of breast tissues can occur from conditions that alter the normal balance of estrogen and androgen levels in the male. Some physiologic changes, medications, and other conditions can cause estrogen levels to rise, or testosterone production or levels to decline. Depending on the causative factor, gynecomastia may be bilateral or unilateral, and can last for a variable length of time.

Causative factors include: (not all inclusive)
- Hormonal imbalance
  - physiologic changes in neonate; at puberty; or at older age
  - hypogonadism: Klinefelter syndrome, testicular neoplasm
  - testicular failure: orchitis, irradiation, trauma
  - endocrine disorder: hyperthyroidism
- Systemic disorders
  - cirrhosis; chronic renal failure; AIDS
- Drug-Medication induced
  - digitalis
  - cimetidine
  - methotrexate,
  - anabolic steroids
  - DHEA, pregnenolone
  - estrogen therapy for prostate cancer
  - marijuana
  - antidepressants
- Estrogen proucing neoplasm
  - testicular
  - hepatoma
  - bronchogenic
  - adrenal
- Idiopathic

Physiologic gynecomastia can occur in the neonate (related to increased estrogen levels from residual maternal hormones); in boys around puberty (from increased free testosterone levels; high estradiol levels); or in elderly men (when testosterone levels decline). Pubertal gynecomastia is most common and affects up to 60% of young males. Physiologic gynecomastia is often bilateral and transient, although it may persist in an elderly man.

The clinical and imaging features of gynecomastia are variable. Unilateral breast enlargement can be worrisome for mass pathology, infection or malignancy and typically undergoes mammographic and/or sonographic evaluation. In some cases, bilateral gynecomastia can be asymmetric and falsely present clinically as only unilateral changes. The early phase of gynecomastia is characterized by proliferation and hyperplasia of the ductal epithelium and myoepithelium. Late changes include the deposition of dense, collagenous, periductal fibrous tissue.

Clinical features of gynecomastia:
• Bilateral or unilateral breast enlargement
• Subareolar thickening, or
• Palpable, firm, subareolar tender lump

Mammographic features:
• (Early) subareolar nodular area of increased density (water-density)
• (Late) fan-shaped radiodense tissue radiating out from nipple
• Diffuse glandular pattern like female breast
• Increase in subcutaneous fat
• No associated calcifications

Sonographic features:
• Hypoechoic, subareolar nodular pattern
• Hypoechoic-to-hyperechoic triangular-shaped region extending from nipple into breast core
• Prominent hypoechoic subareolar ducts surrounded by hyperechoic periductal fibrous tissue
• Possible fluid within duct lumen
• Increase in subcutaneous fat

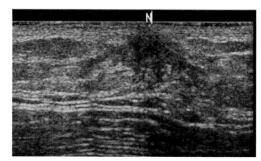 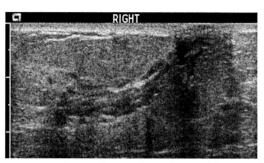

Sonograms of gynecomastia. (Left) Gynecomastia appearing as hypoechoic subareolar nodule with ducts extending into breast core. (Right) Gyncomastia with ductal structures radiating out toward UOQ.

Scanning from a straight anterior approach over the nipple can make subareolar changes appear more mass-like since the ducts are oriented parallel to the sound beam and not well resolved. Using specialized maneuvers (e.g.; two-handed peripheral compression; spatial compound imaging) that align the sound beam more perpendicular to the ducts will allow better demonstratation of ductal changes. In some cases, Doppler may reveal increased flow along the duct wall.

Clinical history is helpful since gynecomastia can mimic inflammation or carcinoma on imaging examinations. Needle biopsy is often necessary to make a definitive diagnosis. Typically, gynecomastia will resolve after the causative factor has been treated or eliminated. Delayed treatment can result in only partial involution of findings.

Pseudogynecomastia is breast enlargement that results from an increased deposition of subcutaneous fat and is bilateral. This is common in obese males and does not involve proliferation of the ductal structures.

D. Male Breast Cancer

Male breast cancer represents less than 1% of all breast malignancies.

Breast cancer usually presents at an older age in men (mean: 64 years) than in women. Since screening mammography is not performed, male breast cancer is usually symptomatic and invasive at time of clinical presentation.

Risk factors include: (not limited to)
- Advanced age
- Exposure to ionizing radiation
- Cryptorchidism
- Testicular injury
- Klinefelter syndrome
- Cowden's syndrome
- Mumps orchitis
- Family history of breast cancer
- Chronic diseases (cirrhosis; AIDS; malnutrition)

Severe and prolonged elevation of the estradial-to-testosterone ratio in a male is a key factor increasing cancer risk. Breast cancer is likely unrelated to gynecomastia, although gynecomastia often co-exists. There is a higher incidence of breast cancer reported in Jewish men.

Histologic types:
- Invasive ductal carcinoma, NOS ($\geq 85\%$)
- DCIS; Paget's disease; Papillary (intraductal/intracystic)
- Sarcoma (4%) including lymphoma
- Other types (Lobular carcinoma is rare since lobule formation is uncommon.)

Clinical features:
- Palpable, hard lump; usually painless
- Subareolar location most common, just eccentric to nipple
- Nipple and skin retraction; possible ulceration
- Possible nipple discharge; often bloody or serosanguinous

Male breast cancer occurs most often in the subareolar region, slightly eccentric to the nipple, and less often in the upper outer quadrant. Cancer is more likely to develop within the central ducts rather than peripherally. Imaging features of malignancy are usually similar to those seen in women for the same cell type. Palpable axillary lymph nodes are common at time of presentation.

Pegasus Lectures, Inc.

Mammographic features:
- Spiculated or angular mass; but may be circumscibed from circumscribed-to-spiculated or angular
- Microcalcifications (30%)
- Subareolar location; eccentric to nipple

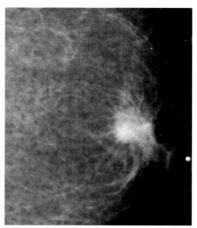

Mammogram of poorly-circumscribed subareolar invasive ductal cancer just eccentric to the nipple.

Sonographic features:
- Round or oval shape
- May be taller-than-wide
- Spiculated or angular mass; thick echogenic halo; shadowing
- May present as circumscribed, hypoechoic mass
- Occasionally complex appearing if central necrosis or intracystic cancer with sound enhancement

Doppler often shows vacularity within the mass. A carcinoma may mimic nodular gynecomastia. A complex lesion may mimic abscess. Biopsy or FNAB is needed to differentiate worrisome lesions.

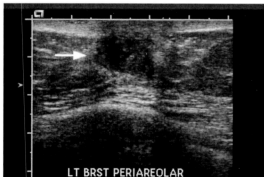

Male breast carcinoma; Intermediate-grade IDC NOS

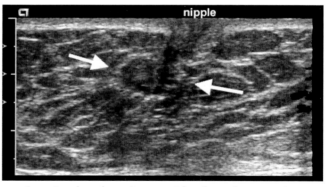

Invasive ductal carcinoma with subareolar extension.

E. Male Breast Metastases

Approximately 0.5-2% of cancers of the male breast are metastatic rather than primary. These include:
- Prostate (most common)
- Melanoma
- Lymphoma
- Lung
- Bladder

• CHAPTER TEN •

Related Diagnostic Examinations
MRI, Sentinel Node Procedure, Ductography and Histology

A. Magnetic Resonance Imaging (M.R.I.)

MRI is a non-ionizing technique that uses a large, powerful magnet to cause hydrogen atoms of the body to give off radio frequency waves. A computer creates a landscape image of the breast from the received radio frequencies. Special breast coils are used for prone breast imaging. Double breast coils allows both breasts to be imaged simultaneously at comparative levels.

Utility of MRI in breast imaging:
- Breast cancer detection
  - High-risk patient with radiographic dense breast and equivocal mammogram or sonogram
  - High-risk patient with positive BRCA1, BRCA2 or other genetic predisposition
  - Identification of site of primary breast cancer in patient with positive axillary lymph nodes and negative or equivocal mammogram or sonogram.
- Staging and treatment planning
  - Determination of multifocal, multicentric, bilateral disease
  - Determination of lymph node involvement
- Evaluation of implant integrity
- Evaluating tumor response to chemotherapy
- Differentiation of tumor recurrence from scar

Limitations in breast imaging:
- Expensive in comparison to mammography and sonography
- Limited number of facilities have breast coils
- Benign mass can show contrast-enhancement and mimic cancer, which lowers sensitivity
- Less effective at detecting lower-grade DCIS.

1. Malignancy
- Mass characterization is based on both morphologic and dynamic (blood flow enhancement) features.
- Cancers are associated with an increase in tumor-related blood flow (neoangiogenesis) and vessel permeability, which causes tumor enhancement on MRI.
- Most invasive tumors show rapid, moderate-to-marked tumor enhancement following IV injection of a paramagnetic contrast agent (Gadolinium), with subsequent contrast wash out. A rim-enhancing lesion is very suggestive of cancer.
- Contrast-enhanced MRI is the most sensitive supplemental imaging modality for breast cancer detection. Specificity is better in high-risk patients since some benign processes show contrast enhancement.
- *In 2007, the American Cancer Society published recommendations for screening MRI as an adjunct to mammography that included women with an approximately 20-25% chance or greater lifetime risk of breast cancer.*

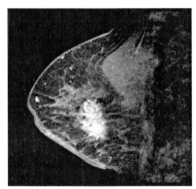

Contrast-enhanced MRI Breast Cancer

2. **Staging and Treatment Planning**
   - Contrast-enhanced MRI is very sensitive at detecting primary invasive carcinomas, additional tumor foci, and nodal involvement which helps determine the extent of disease.
   - Mammography is limited to seeing lower axillary nodes. MRI can detect involvement of level I-III, internal mammary and supraclavicular nodes.
   - Features worrisome for nodal metastases include:
     - enhancement on contrast-enhanced study
     - nodal enlargement and fixation to surrounding tissues

3. **Implant Integrity**
   - Non-enhanced MRI is the most accurate modality for evaluating implants for rupture.
   - MRI is especially effective at evaluating double-lumen implants for failure because reflections from the internal implant chamber can potentially mimic intracapsular rupture on a sonogram
   - MRI features of intracapsular silicone rupture include:
     - "Linguine" or "wavy-line" sign represents collapsed elastomer shell suspended within silicone contained by the fibrous capsule. The infolded implant shell appears as low signal, overlapping curvilinear structure within the high signal silicone gel (T2-weighted, fast spin echo, water suppression images).
     - "Teardrop" or "noose" sign indicates uncollapsed rupture with silicone gel trapped inside a peripheral (radial) fold. The "keyhole" sign also refers to silicone inside and outside a radial fold.
   - MRI features of extracapsular rupture
     - MRI is effective at determining the presence, amount, and location of soft-tissue silicone.
     - Silicone granuloma appears as hyperintense tissue outside the fibrous capsule on T2-weighted images with water suppression and hypointense on T1-weighted images with silicone suppression.
   - MRI can detect silicone within lymph nodes
   - MRI is more sensitive at detecting silicone fluid /gel bleed

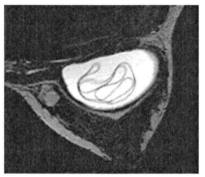

MRI Silicone implant: Intracapsular rupture
Courtesy   Michael Middleton, MD

B. Ductography

Ductography and galactography are terms used to describe the radiographic examination of the lactiferous ducts using a radiopaque, contrast agent. A water-soluble, iodinated contrast agent is used to reduce the incidence of duct irritation.

Ductography is often the procedure of choice for examining the patient with clinically worrisome nipple discharge. Ductography is performed to determine the cause of the nipple discharge and also to localize the affected duct prior to surgery. Although nipple discharge is an indication for breast sonography, some intraductal masses or wall proliferations are too small to be detected on a sonogram. However, sonography can often detect large duct papillary lesions and provide an alternative to diagnostic galactography. If an intraductal mass is detected by sonography, US-guided core biopsy can be performed.

Ductography Indications - Contraindications:
*   The primary indication for ductography is abnormal, spontaneous nipple discharge from a single duct. (The most common cause of pathologic discharge is a papilloma. In such cases, the discharge will be bloody, serous or clear.)
*   Ductography is contraindicated in patients with mastitis, iodinated contrast allergy or nipple surgery.

Description of Ductography Procedure:
*   Nipple discharge allows identification of the duct orifice for retrograde injection of approximately 1cc of contrast using a 27 to 30-g sialography needle.
*   (Sonography can guide placement of a 25-g needle into a dilated subareolar duct for contrast injection when nipple cannulation fails.)
*   After contrast injection, a series of mammographic C-C and 90^0 lateral images are taken to show the ductal system. Opacification of the duct allows evaluation of duct dilatation, internal filling defects, and duct irregularity.

Findings:
*   A normal opacified duct is typically smooth-walled and tapers in size within the breast core.
*   A solitary papilloma can appear as a focal, intraductal filling defect; can be the cause of duct expansion, irregularity, or distortion.
*   With fibrocystic change, there may be duct dilatation and wall irregularity. Opacified cysts or cyst clusters may be seen communicating within terminal duct lobular units.
*   Cancer causes filling defects, abrupt cut-off at the mass site, or duct displacement or irregularity.

Air bubbles can simulate intraductal filling defects but typically shift in position between views.

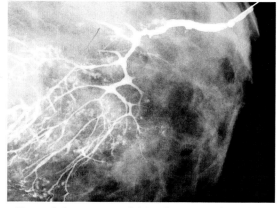

Normal ductogram of ductal system of one lobe.

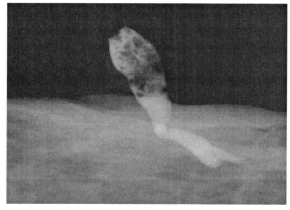

Filling defect from nipple adenoma.
(Courtesy: Cindy Rapp, BS, RDMS)

Saline-infusion ultrasound ductography can help distend a subareolar duct for enhanced demonstration of intraductal lesions.

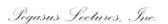

C. Sentinel Lymph Node Biopsy Procedure

The first node to receive lymphatic drainage from a primary breast cancer is at most risk for metastasis. This node is called the sentinel node. The sentinel node is typically an axillary lymph node.

In the past, complete axillary lymph node dissection (ALND) was routinely performed in breast cancer patients. Unfortunately, this procedure has a high incidence of complications that includes arm lymphedema, nerve damage, and potential loss of arm and shoulder function. To reduce the morbidity associated with complete ALND, many surgeons now prefer to perform a sentinel node biopsy and remove much fewer axillary nodes if shown to be cancer free.

Lymphoscintigraphy is a nuclear medicine procedure that uses a radioisotope to map lymphatic flow from a primary breast cancer to the first draining lymph node in the lymphatic basin. Using this technique, the sentinel node can be identified for biopsy in patients without clinically suspicious axillary nodes.

Lymphoscintigraphy - Sentinel Node Biopsy Procedure:
*   The radioactive agent (typically technetium-99m-labeled filtered sulfur colloid mixed with saline) is injected in front of the breast tumor and/or in the periareolar region. If needed, sonography can guide injection adjacent to the tumor. Over a period of time, the radioactive agent flows through the lymphatics and concentrates in the sentinel node.
*   The concentrated isotope creates a "hot spot" on the nuclear medicine scan that identifies the location of the sentinel node.
*   In the operating room, the surgeon can inject blue dye near the tumor as an additional mapping agent.
*   A gamma probe (scintillation counter) is used to locate the radioactive node for removal and biopsy. Blue dye will also be contained within the node.
*   The sentinel node is removed and examined by the pathologist to determine if cancer cells are present. (In some facilities, ultrasound is used to biopsy or localize the sentinel node in the operating room prior to removal.)

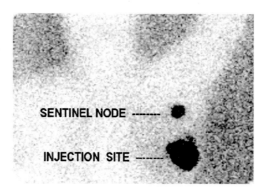

Lymphoscintigraphy shows location of axillary sentinel node prior to biopsy

If the node is tumor free, the patient may be spared a complete axillary lymph node dissection. A negative sentinel node procedure has a 95-100% likelihood of representing a clear axillary nodal basin.

Sparing the patient a complete ALND is desired to reduce complications and to preserve arm function.

Sonography can be used to evaluate and to biopsy suspicious axillary lymph nodes in patients with suspected or known breast cancer. If the axillary node is positive for cancer cells, lymphoscintigraphy with sentinel node biopsy is not usually performed and a more extensive ALND is warranted.

D. Histology

Histology is the microscopic study of tissue. Histopathology is the microscopic study of diseased tissue. Histologic analysis includes the minute structure, composition, and function of tissues.

Histologic analysis differentiates normal tissue from physiological changes or from pathologic disease. Histologic differentiation of cancer is based on the types and patterns of cells and the effects on surrounding tissue.

For example, histologic analysis can differentiate:
- benign vs. malignant disease
- in situ vs. invasive carcinoma
- ductal vs. lobular carcinoma
- proliferative vs. involutional changes
- secretory vs. proliferative menstrual changes
- stromal vs. epithelial tissue

Major histologic types of breast cancer include:

- ductal carcinoma in situ	- invasive ductal, NOS
- lobular carcinoma in situ	- invasive lobular carcinoma
- papillary carcinoma in situ	- invasive papillary carcinoma
- Paget's disease	- tubular carcinoma
- medullary carcinoma	- mucinous carcinoma

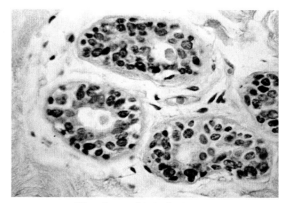
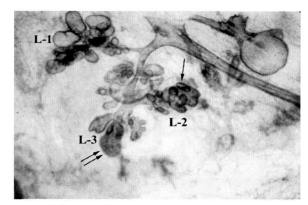

Histology of lobule / acini   *Subgross photograph of lobular changes*
(http://mammary.nih.gov.com)

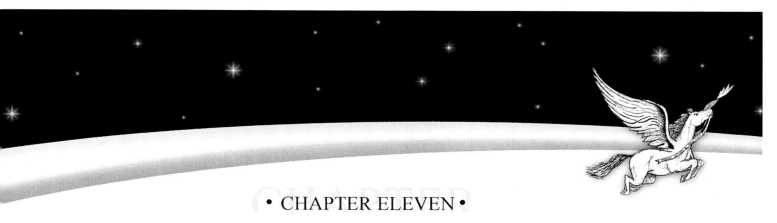

• CHAPTER ELEVEN •

Breast Implants

A. Indications for Implants and Placement Sites

Indications
Mammary implants are used for the following reasons:
* Cosmetic augmentation (most common)
* Post-mastectomy reconstruction
* Congenital amastia
* Severe hypoplasia or asymmetry
* Inlays for tissue defects

Approximately 60-80% of implant surgeries are for cosmetic augmentation. The most common "medical" reason for implants is post-mastectomy reconstruction.

Sites of Implant Placement
* Subglandular   (submammary; prepectoral)
* Submuscular   (subpectoral; retropectoral)
* (Subcutaneous)
* (Intramammary)

For cosmetic augmentation mammoplasty, implants are typically placed beneath the glandular tissue (subglandular), in front of the pectoralis major muscle.

A submuscular location is typical for post-mastectomy reconstruction. Implant placement beneath the pectoralis muscle in patients with augmentation mammoplasty allows easier evaluation of the breast tissue during mammography. A subpectoral location lowers the incidence of capsular contracture, but can be subject to implant migration.

A subcutaneous, prepectoral location is an alternative placement site for post-mastectomy reconstruction and for tissue expanders.

Routes for implant placement can be periareolar, inframammary, axillary, or through a paraumbilical incision.

Intramammary implants are used for tissue inlays.

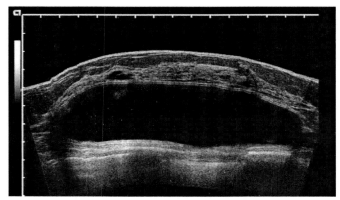

Subglandular saline implant – singe lumen;
Breast augmentation

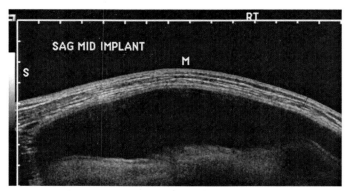

Submuscular silicone implant – single lumen;
Post-mastectomy breast reconstruction

Note:

In some augmentation patients, the inferior portion of a subpectoral implant may partially extend to a subglandular location (in front of the serratus anterior muscle) because the pectoralis major muscle thins and tapers inferiorly. However, the pectoralis muscle will amply cover the superior portion of the implant. Scanning the upper outer segment of the implant near the axilla will allow correct identification of the implant as being submuscular in location.

B. **Types of Breast Implants - Prostheses**
There are over 200 different types and variations of breast implants.

Common types of breast implants include:
- Saline-filled; single-lumen (most common implant in current use)
- Silicone types
  - Single-lumen gel filled
  - Double-lumen
    - outer saline lumen; inner silicone lumen
    - outer silicone lumen; inner saline lumen
- Saline-inflatable tissue expanders (following mastectomy)

Autologous (donor tissue) reconstruction:
- Transverse rectus abdominis muscle (TRAM) flap
- Latissimus dorsi flap

Single lumen implants contain either saline or silicone gel. Most silicone implants are single-lumen, gel-filled. The most common double-lumen implant has an inner silicone chamber surrounded by an outer saline chamber. Filling ports or valves are found with expandable saline implants or chambers.

The elastomer or polyurethane shell of an implant can be smooth or textured. Texturing helps to reduce fibrous scarring around the implant.

Silicone gel implants are generally preferred because of their more natural feel and appearance and often less prone to traumatic rupture than saline implants. In 1992, the U.S. Food and Drug Administration (FDA) restricted the use of silicone gel implants for cosmetic augmentation because of health concerns related to leakage. The FDA still allowed silicone implants for reconstructive mammoplasty. In late 2006, the FDA deemed silicone-gel implants to be safe and effective after extensive clinical studies and re-approved their use with minor restrictions. Manufacturers are now required to conduct a post-approval study to monitor silicone implant patients for a period of ten years.

Direct injection of silicone, paraffin, or fat for breast augmentation is no longer practiced. Direct silicone injections caused severe complications and granuloma formation. The placement of polyvinyl sponges for augmentation has also been discontinued.

Autologous Reconstruction

Transverse rectus abdominis muscle (TRAM) flap procedure is a form of autologous tissue transplantation for breast reconstruction following mastectomy. A section of the periumbilical abdominal wall and subcutaneous fat, along with the associated muscular and vascular pedicles, is transferred to the breast. With a "free flap" procedure, there is complete removal of the donor tissue, which is reattached to the breast by microsurgery.

A latissimus dorsi flap procedure involves transfer of tissue (muscle, fat, skin) from the upper back to the breast region.

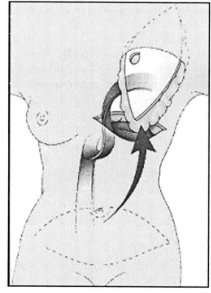

Tram flap reconstruction.
(Modified from: LePage M et al;
Breast reconstruction with TRAM flaps:
Normal and abnormal appearances at CT.
Radiographics. 1999;19:1593-1603.)

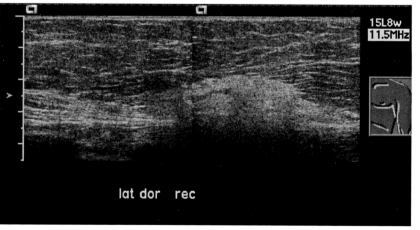

Latissimus dorsi flap; partial reconstruction.

C. Implant Complications
Complications related to breast implants can occur shortly, or months to years following implantation.

Breast Implant Complications:

Short-term (Acute)	Long-Term (Chronic)
• Pain and tenderness • Bleeding - Hematoma • Infection - Abscess • Seroma • Loss of nipple sensation	• Capsular fibrosis/calcification • Capsular Contracture • Herniation • Migration • Chronic infection • Rupture • Silicone granuloma

1. Fibrous capsule
A thin rim of scar tissue (fibrous capsule) commonly forms around a breast implant, adjacent to the outer shell. Fibrous encapsulation is the most common implant comlplication. Scarring begins within weeks of implantation.

Formation of the fibrous capsule is the body's normal response to the presence of a foreign body, and is most apparent with silicone implants. The elastomer shell of a silicone implant is semi-permeable. Over a period of time, microscopic amounts of silicone fluid can seep through the intact membrane to its outer surface. This "silicone gel bleed" can accentuate fibrous scarring, and increase the risk of contracture. Since the 1980s, fluorsilicone has been added to the elastomer shell to reduce permeability.

2. Capsular Contracture
Hardening and distortion of an implant occurs when there is tightening and constriction of the surrounding fibrous capsule. Capsular contracture causes the implant to become more rounded or balloon-shaped, thereby causing breast asymmetry or distortion. Capsular contracture more often affects subglandular silicone implants. Closed capsulotomy preformed to reduce capsular contracture can increase the risk of implant herniation and rupture.

Thin, smooth implant shells are more prone to severe fibrous encapsulation and rupture. A fibrous capsule exceeding 1.5mm in thickness is reported to be associated with capsular contracture. Texturing of the implant shell, the application of a polyurethane coating, and/or subpectoral implant placement helps to reduce the amount of fibrous scarring and contracture. Textured implants have a thicker shell that helps reduce the incidence of rupture. Most single-lumen implants used since the 1980's have textured surfaces.

Methods to Reduce Risk of Implant Capsular Contracture
Subpectoral implant placement
Use of saline implants
Texturing of implant shell
Adding fluorsilicone to elastomer shell
Adding polyurethane to textured shell
No longer recommended: Closed capsulectomy

Textured, polyurethane-coated implants may demonstrate a thin amount of serous fluid between the outer implant shell and the fibrous capsule. This small implant effusion is not an indication of rupture. Instead, the fluid provides a thin space for the implant to move and maintain its flexibility.

3. Capsular Calcification

Over time, calcification may develop along the fibrous capsule. This feature can be seen on a mammogram along the implant surface. On a sonogram, extensive calcification can cause sound attenuation that limits implant evaluation.

4. Herniation

A localized break in the fibrous capsule can allow a portion of an intact implant to bulge through the opening. Herniation of the implant may cause a palpable abnormality. Sonography and MRI are effective at detecting implant herniation. At times, mammography may have difficulty differentiating herniation from extracapsular rupture.

5. Rupture

Rupture is the second most common complication and is classified as intracapsular or as extracapsular. Intracapsular rupture can be minimal or involve complete infolding of the implant shell. (See separate sections on imaging findings of rupture.) Besides trauma, implant age is a key risk factor for rupture. The detection of silicone-gel implant rupture is of more medical significance since extruded silicone can cause an inflammatory response leading to granuloma formation. Most silicone implants show some degree of implant rupture by 11-15 years.

Rupture of a saline prosthesis results in implant deflation with absorption of the saline by the body. Saline implant deflation is apparent clinically and does not require imaging. However, mammography, as well as sonography, can easily confirm this finding.

D. Normal Implants - Sonographic Appearance

Sonographic features of a normal single-lumen breast implant include:

Saline - Single-lumen	Silicone Gel - Single-lumen
• Defined implant shell / tissue interface • Smooth contour, elliptical shape • Anechoic lumen • Anterior reverberation	• Defined implant shell /tissue interface • Smooth contour, elliptical shape • Anechoic lumen, low-level echoes at higher gain • Anterior reverberation
Additional findings: • Actual size = US size • Filling valve • Possible peripheral fold	Additional findings: • Propagation speed artifact (AP size > Actual) • Possible peripheral fold

The inner and outer surfaces of the implant shell can be resolved with high frequency transducers and appear as two highly echogenic, thin, parallel-lines. The echo-poor area between these lines represents the thickness of the implant shell. Depending on the resolution of the transducer, the fibrous capsule may be seen abutting the outer surface of the implant shell, giving it a 3-line appearance. On a sonogram, the outer surface of a smooth-walled implant shell will be more distinct than a textured implant shell. A small amount of pericapsular fluid may occur with polyurethane covered or textured implants, which can mimic implant leakage.

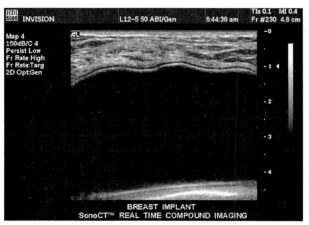

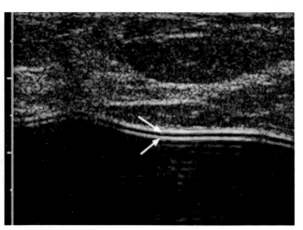

Saline implant; Subglandular placement
Mild wrinkling of anterior implant surface
(Courtesy: Philips Medical Systems)

Non-textured elastomer shell: Arrows point
to 2 parallel, echogenic lines that represent
the outer and inner walls of the implant shell.

A diaphragm-type fill port or expander valve is commonly seen along the anterior surface of a saline implant or a tissue expander. Double lumen implants also have valves that allow expansion of the saline chamber. Filling valves are often located beneath the areola. However, the position of the valve can shift due to implant migration or capsular contracture. Ports or valve may become palpable when there is little overlying tissue.

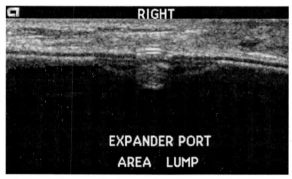

Saline implant: Expander port – Discoid Fill valve

A radial (peripheral) fold is a normal finding and not an implant complication. A peripheral fold extends from the inner wall for a variable distance within the implant. Fluid or silicone gel outside the implant shell can potentially accumulate within the fold. Internal long, wavy, or complex folds can simulate a double lumen or implant rupture.

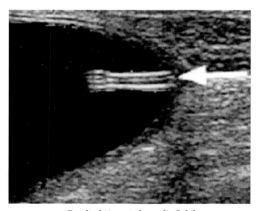

Radial (peripheral) fold

142

Folding or wrinkling of the implant shell can occur secondary to implant contracture by fibrous encapsulation, from placement within a small insertion pocket, or from underfilling of the implant. Implant wrinkles causes lobulation of the implant shell; however, the elastomer shell maintains close apposition to the fibrous capsule. Saline implants are more prone to wrinkling and folding.

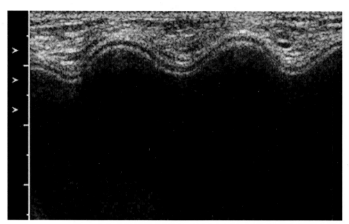

Implant wrinkles seen in close apposition to fibrous shell.

Reverberation artifact is commonly seen as repeating bands of echoes along the anterior margin of the implant where the sound beam is perpendicular to the implant. This artifact is often more pronounced with silicone implants.

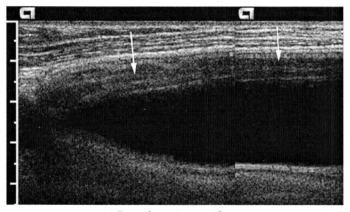

Reverberation artifact

Lighter scanning pressure, or the use of tissue harmonic imaging or compound imaging, will help to reduce reveberation artifact. Reverberation artifact can reduce sensitivity at detecting intracapsular rupture.

A propagation speed artifact is seen with silicone implants that helps to identify the implant type. The speed of sound through silicone (~1000m/s) is slower than through soft tissue (1540m/s) or saline. Since the ultrasound system assumes a propagation speed of 1540 m/s, echoes from structures deep to a silicone implant arrive later than expected and are, therefore, artifactually depicted deeper than in reality. This depth distortion makes the AP dimension of the implant appear larger than its actual size on the ultrasound image. When scanning along the edge of the implant by the chest wall, there will be a "step-down" or "step off" of the chest wall echoes beneath the implant. For double-lumen implants with an internal silicone chamber, the step-down effect will occur beneath the silicone, rather than the saline, chamber.

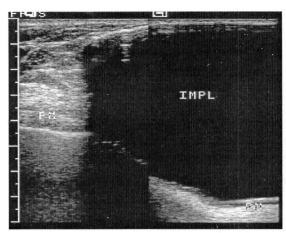

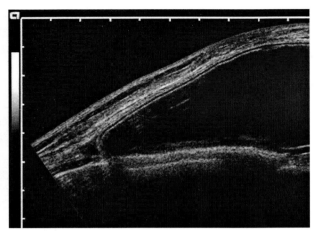

Silicone implant: Propagation speed artifact.
Slower speed of sound though silicone causes
"step-off" effect of chest wall beneath the implant

Saline implant with no "step-off" effect
of the chest wall beneath the implant

To fully penetrate the breast tissue and implant may require reducing the transducer frequency from 10-12 MHz to 5-7 MHz. Special techniques such as EFOV imaging, split-screen (dual-mode) imaging, or use of a convex-linear or curved-array transducer can better show the size and contour of the implant. Spit-screen imaging also allows comparative scanning of the right and left breasts at similar levels.

During scanning, special attention should be paid to the edges of the implant shell, which are often thinner and more prone to rupture.

Dynamic compression can help compare the compressibility of each implant when assessing hardening from capsular contracture.

E. Silicone Implant Rupture

1. Intracapsular Rupture
The majority of silicone implant ruptures are intracapsular. Trauma and advancing age of the prosthesis increases the risk of implant failure. With intracapsular rupture (ICR), silicone gel leaks outside of the implant through a defect in the elastomer shell but is still contained by the fibrous capsule. Ultrasound findings are most reliable when there is significant collapse and infolding of the implant.

Main Sonographic Features of Intracapsular Silicone Implant Rupture

US Finding	Description
"Stepladder" or " Parallel-line" sign (most reliable finding)	Multiple, parallel, echogenic, linear bands reflecting from overlapping, infolded layers of the collapsed implant shell that is suspended in silicone gel contained by the fibrous capsule.
Increased echogenicity of silicone gel (focal, globular, diffuse) (suspicious, but not definitive finding)	A tear in the implant shell can allow mixing of silicone with body fluids, proteins, and organic salts, which can cause an increase in silicone echogenicity.

Less definitive findings include: focal or irregular implant bulge; poorly-defined implant margin; or short, discontinuous internal parallel lines.

The "stepladder" or "parallel-line" sign associated with ICR on a sonogram correlates with the "linguine" or "wavy-line" sign seen on a MRI exam. (Unenhanced MRI is the most accurate imaging modality for assessing implant integrity. MRI is especially effective at evaluating double-lumen implants for failure because reflections from the internal implant chamber can potentially mimic intracapsular rupture on a sonogram.)

Conventional linear array imaging demonstrates infolded implant layers that are parallel to the transducer face (perpendicular to the sound beam). 3-D or spatial compounding techniques may better show the curved edges of a collapsed implant.

A small amount of silicone entrapped by a radial fold has a "noose-like" (ie, keyhole-, teardrop-, noose sign) appearance on MRI and US. This finding can also be seen with uncollapsed rupture. A hematoma or seroma between the fibrous capsule and implant shell can simulate implant rupture.

Pockets of material previously injected into the silicone gel at the time of implantation (saline, antibiotics, providone-iodine, steroids) to help reduce infection and fibrous encapsulation can cause the silicone within an intact implant to appear more echogenic and heterogeneous. Such an imaging pattern can make the interpretation of ICR more difficult.

On a mammogram, silicone is radiopaque and obscures ICR detection.

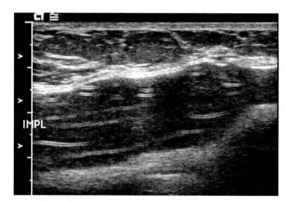 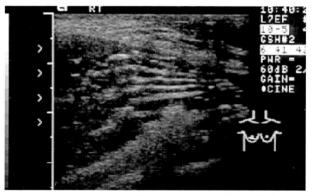

Intracapsular silicone implant rupture: Examples of the ultrasound demonstration of "stepladder" or "parallel-track" sign

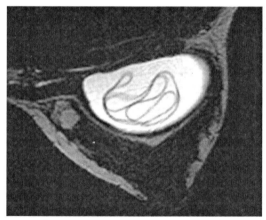

Non-enhanced MRI of intracapsular rupture: Demonstration of "linguini" sign representing infolded implant floating in silicone contained by the fibrous capsule (Courtesy: M. Middleton, MD)

2. Extracapsular Rupture

Extracapsular rupture (ECR) indicates leakage of silicone gel through a breach in the implant shell AND the fibrous capsule. ECR allows migration of silicone into the breast tissue, along the chest wall, and to distant sites.

Main Sonographic Features of Extracapsular Silicone Implant Rupture

US Finding	Description
"Echogenic Noise" or "Snowstorm" Sign (most predictive finding)	These terms describe the characteristic sonographic appearance of microglobules of silicone within soft tissue or lymph nodes. Affected tissues appear highly echogenic with "dirty shadowing" that obscures posterior structures. This pattern may result from the marked variation in acoustic properties at the tissue/silicone interfaces.
Hypoechoic or anechoic fluid collection or globule outside the fibrous capsule (silicone fluid/gel) (less predictive finding)	A collection of free silicone gel or silicone globule may be seen outside the capsule, and must be differentiated from other fluid collections or cysts. Echogenic noise often surrounds a silicone globule.

Indeterminate findings include: implant bulge, peri-implant fluid collection

The presence of extracapsular silicone is quickly walled off by an inflammatory response and forms a silicone granuloma.

Typically, sonographic signs of ICR accompany ECR. Patient history is important since residual silicone can be present in patients with a prior history of implant rupture and interval implant replacement.

The presence of "echogenic noise" is not always conclusive for ECR. Occasionally, very small areas of "echogenic noise" are located at the margin of intact-appearing implant. It is reported that small amounts of silicone fluid can "bleed" through a porous, although otherwise intact implant. Since silicone can be taken up by the lymphatic system, some lymph nodes may display "echogenic noise."

Care must be taken not to confuse normal, small periimplant effusions for ECR when no significant intracapsular findings are present.

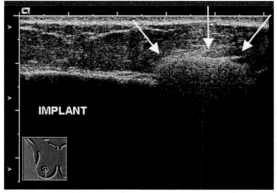

Extracapsular rupture: US demonstration of "echogenic noise" indicating silicone in tissues outside the fibrous capsule.

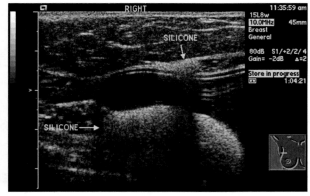

Demonstration of residual silicone in a prior silicone implant rupture and replacement with saline implants.

Pegasus Lectures, Inc.

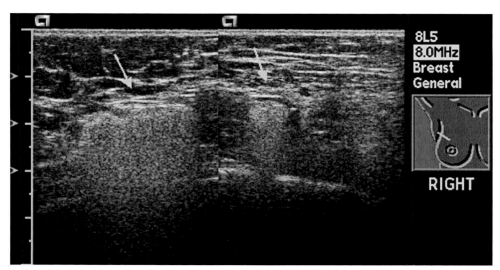

Demonstration of "echogenic noise" within axillary lymph nodes in a patient with subpectoral silicone implant rupture.

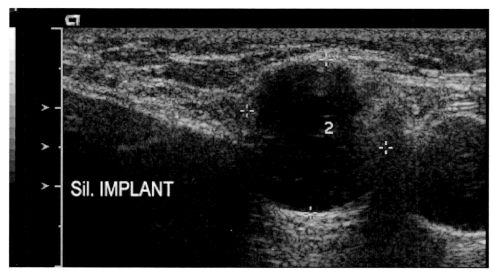

Extruded silicone gel globules with cyst-like appearance.

F. Mammographic Implant Evaluation

Mammography can verify the placement site of an implant. Saline is less dense on a mammogram than silicone, thereby allowing detection of some internal folds and filling ports. Additionally, mammography can differentiate the internal silicone chamber of a double lumen implant from the outer saline chamber. At times, mammography can also tell if the implant has a smooth or a textured surface.

Saline obscures less adjacent breast tissues than silicone. Silicone is impenetrable by x-ray and disallows examination of the internal contents or underlying tissues. Therefore, mammography is not effective at diagnosing intracapsular rupture of a single lumen, silicone-gel implant. However, mammography can help detect capsular calcification, as well as extracapsular silicone that projects away from the implant on specific mammographic views. However, the opacity of silicone can make it difficult to differentiate herniation from rupture when there is a focal irregularity or bulge in continuity with the implant surface.

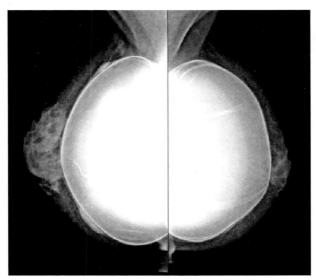

MLO mammograms demonstrating bilateral subglandular saline implants.

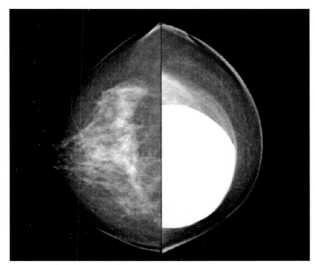

CC mammogram of left subpectoral silicone implant.

Special "pushback" or Eklund views allow exclusion of the implant on the mammogram for better evaluation of the breast tissue. However, even with specialty views, implants can obscure a significant portion of the breast tissue. Therefore, sonography plays an important role in the evaluation of breast tissue that may be suboptimally evaluated by mammography.

• CHAPTER TWELVE •

Ultrasound-Guided Interventional Procedures

A. Indications

In many facilities, sonography has become the modality of choice for guidance during interventional procedures of ultrasound detectable masses. Compared to stereotactic-guidance, ultrasound is faster, often less expensive, and usually more comfortable for patients.

Breast interventional procedures can be:
*   Diagnostic
*   Therapeutic

Conventional indications for ultrasound guidance include:
*   Aspiration of certain complicated, complex, or symptomatic cysts
*   Biopsy of indeterminate or suspicious solid mass
*   Biopsy of a suspicious lymph node
*   Drainage of abscess, hematoma, or persistent seroma
*   Pre-operative dye and/or wire localization of a nonpalpable mass

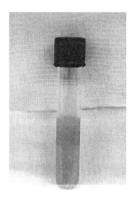
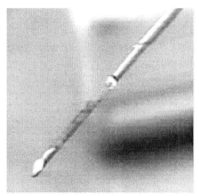

Cyst aspirate for cytologic analysis.   *Tissue core for histologic analysis.*

Newer applications for ultrasound guidance include:
*   Radioisotope and/or dye injection for sentinel node biopsy procedure
*   Contrast or saline injection into duct for galactography when duct orifice cannot be cannulated
*   Radiofrequency tumor ablation
*   Post biopsy clip marker placement
*   Implantation of metallic markers in tumor bed of patient receiving preoperative chemotherapy
*   Intraoperative localization of silicone or of a nonpalpable mass

Additionally, sonography can provide post-operative specimen examination.

B. Advantages - Disadvantages of Ultrasound-guided Interventional Procedures

Advantages of US-guidance include:
- Real-time visualization of anesthesia injection
- Real-time visualization of needle approach to the mass
- Visual confirmation of needle sampling of the mass
- Documentation of complete evacuation of cystic mass
- Ability to biopsy a mass located close to the chest wall
- Ability to biopsy a mass seen on only one radiographic view
- Ability to detect blood flow around or within the mass
- More choices in patient positioning
- Usually more comfortable for patient than prone stereotactic or MRI biopsy
- Often faster than x-ray stereotactic or MRI biopsy
- Often less expensive than stereotactic procedure or MRI biopsy

Disadvantages of US-Guidance include:
- Limited ability to visualize and sample suspicious microcalcifications
- Limited stabilization of tissues in large-breasted patient

C. Guidance Methods

There are a variety of methods can be used to guide needle or catheter placement during breast interventional procedures.

Physicians performing interventional procedure most often prefer the "free-hand technique". With this method, the physician typically holds the transducer in one hand while simultaneously advancing the needle toward the mass during real-time observation. When desired, the sonographer holds the transducer during imaging, while the physician manipulates the needle. The obliquity at which the needle is advanced toward the mass affects how well the needle shaft and tip is demonstrated during real-time imaging.

1. Free-hand technique:
- Near-vertical approach
  - Allows needle placement over the shortest path to the mass
  - Needle placed alongside mid portion of long-axis of transducer
  - Needle is directed in a near-vertical path toward mass
  - Short-axis portion of needle seen within mass
  - Drawback: Steep angle limits needle visualization of shaft/tip

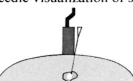

- Oblique path
- "Parallel-to-chest"; "Parallel-to-transducer" technique
  - Needle advanced parallel to transducer face, skin, chest wall under long-axis of transducer (long-axis approach)
  - Maximizes visualization of needle tip and shaft since sound beam is directed perpendicular to needle
  - Reduces risk of pneumothorax when biopsy deep lesion
  - Drawback: longer needle path to mass

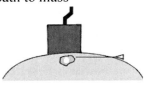

Pegasus Lectures, Inc.

To gain skill at the free-hand technique, physicians are encouraged to practice needle placement using a self-made or commercially available breast biopsy phantom.

Ultrasound-guided aspiration and biopsy procedures are performed on an outpatient basis. This significantly reduces costs when a benign diagnosis obviates the need for surgical excision of a breast mass.

2. **Transducer needle guide:**
   - Preset angle of needle path
   - Drawback: Limits ability to make quick adjustments in needle angulation

Transducer needle-guide attachments are available on most breast systems but are used less often during breast interventional procedures than a free handed technique.

Some newer systems incorporate "virtual needle-guide" technology whereby the projected path of the needle is displayed on the ultrasound monitor without the physical limitations of an attached needle-guide.

D. Steps To a Successful Interventional Procedure
   Steps to a successful interventional procedure are outlined below:
   - Obtain patient history that includes known allergies to topical agents or to medications that will be used during the procedure.
   - Obtain / Review pertinent sonograms and mammograms.
   - Obtain patient consent.
     - Inform patient of interventional procedure
     - Explain possible complications
     - Discuss alternative procedures
   - Prepare appropriate supplies.
   - Utilize sterile technique.
   - Optimize patient positioning.
   - Secure diagnostic specimen by performance of the procedure by a qualified physician with appropriate assistance by a sonographer.
   - Accurately handle, prepare, and label specimen for cytologic or histologic analysis.
   - Provide appropriate post-biopsy patient care; aftercare instructions
   - Receive accurate interpretation of specimen by qualified pathologist or cytopathologist.
   - Have radiologist/surgeon correlate cytology or pathology report with ultrasound findings to verify adequate sampling.
   - Physician may need to repeat biopsy, or recommend excisional biopsy, if histologic findings are not concordant with ultrasound features of lesion.

E. Complications
   Complications related to breast interventional procedures are uncommon but include:
   - Localized pain
   - Bleeding - Hematoma
   - Infection
   - Allergic reaction
   - Pneumothorax
   - Implant rupture

Potential complications should be explained to the patient before the consent form is signed.

Localized pain can be reduced by appropriate technique and administration of a local anesthetic during the procedure. A non-aspirin oral analgesic may be recommended to reduce pain following the procedure.

Patients taking daily aspirin or anticoagulatory medication are at increased risk for hematoma formation. The physician or radiologist may recommend suspending the patient's medication for a limited number of days before the biopsy to reduce the risk of excessive bleeding. Coagulatory laboratory tests can help determine the complication risk. Doppler can be helpful in assessing tumor vascularity before needle insertion. Avoidance of puncturing sizable vessels along the needle path will reduce significant bleeding. In general, bleeding can be minimized by the application of compression over the puncture site following an interventional procedure. Placement of an ice pack or gauze pack between the skin and bra after the procedure can further limit hematoma formation.

Infection is typically eliminated by good sterile technique. However, secondary infection can occur after an interventional procedure from bacteria entering the breast through the puncture site, before it has healed. Providing the patient with appropriate aftercare instructions can help reduce the chance of infection.

Obtaining good patient history can eliminate known allergic reactions to topical agents or anesthetics.

Pneumothorax is more likely to occur from a procedure utilizing a spring-loaded automated biopsy device. If the biopsy needle is fired too steeply at a deeply-located lesion, the needle may puncture the chest wall and cause a pneumothorax. To avoid this complication, the needle should be advanced and fired in a path parallel to the chest wall at the level of the lesion.

Implant rupture is less likely when performing a fine-needle aspiration biopsy, rather than a spring-loaded automated biopsy. Attention must be paid to direct the needle away from the implant margin.

Although percutaneous needle biopsy is less traumatic than excisional biopsy, the sonographer should be aware of acute and chronic changes that can follow certain breast interventional procedures. Breast alterations related to trauma include skin thickening, edema, hematoma, seroma, abscess, cyst infection, fat necrosis, architectural distortion, and scarring. A seroma or hematoma that forms within a mammotomy cavity may take up 3-6 weeks to resolve.

Additional vascular complications related to large core biopsies are arteriovenous fistula and pseudoaneurysm. In some situations, ultrasound-guided thrombin injection is necessary to treat pseudoaneurysms.

F. Cyst Aspiration

Purpose:
- Aspiration of complicated or certain complex cysts*
- Aspiration of symptomatic cyst (e.g., painful, large)
- Aspiration of cyst(s) interfering with clinical or mammographic evaluation
* Complex cystic and solid lesions should undergo biopsy

Additional biopsy or excision may be required when:
- Aspirate is bloody
- Palpable mass does not fully evacuate / resolve after aspiration
- Cyst shows wall thickening, thick septations, or mural nodule
- Cyst recurs within short time period

Cytologic analysis:
- Cytologic analysis to exclude malignant cells (e.g., bloody aspirate)
- Microbiology analysis (culture, Gram stain / sensitivity) is ordered for a cloudy - purulent aspirate to exclude infection

General Procedure Description:
- Performed with/without local anesthetic
- 20-22 gauge needle is attached to a small syringe (with or without connective tubing) and advanced into the dependent portion of the cyst for aspiration. A 16- or 18-gauge needle may be needed to aspirate thicker fluids. Alternatively, a vacutainer device may be used.
- Needle placement and mass evacuation is observed during real-time scanning.
- Injection of an equal amount of air to the amount of fluid aspirated can reduce cyst recurrence.
- Document amount and appearance of aspirated fluid and any complications.
- Note: If grossly bloody aspirate present, consider core or vacuum-assisted biopsy and or clip placement.

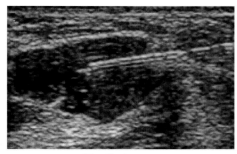
Needle in cyst

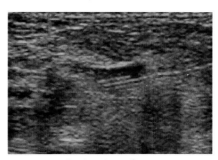
Aspiration of cyst

G. Fine-Needle Aspiration Biopsy (FNAB)

Fine-needle aspiration biopsy (FNAB) allows multidirectional sampling of a breast mass using a small-gauge needle to obtain cellular material for cytologic analysis. This technique is generally used for the diagnostic evaluation of a complex mass, a small solid indeterminate mass, or for lymph node analysis.

Advantages of FNAB compared to other percutaneous biopsy techniques include:
- Lower cost
- Less traumatic; less complications (least traumatic form of biopsy)
- Faster results from cytologic analysis
- Often safer technique for sampling or aspirating mass near implant wall or near chest wall

Disadvantages – Limitations of FNAB include:
- Greater chance of undersampling solid mass. Sampling errors can cause false-negative diagnosis, especially in small fibrous tumors.
- Requires expert cytopathologist to ensure accurate interpretation
- Cytologic specimen does not accurately differentiate in situ from invasive cancers.
- Blood in aspirate can reduce diagnostic accuracy.
- Inappropriate technique for sampling microcalcifications

General Procedure Description:
- 20-22 (or smaller) gauge needle is attached to a 5-10cc syringe or an aspiration gun
- Needle is advanced to the mass under real-time US-guidance
- Multiple back-and-forth and multidirectional passes are made within the mass while suction is applied
- Aspirate is placed on glass slides, fixed, and sent for microscopic, cytologic analysis

The failure of cytologic analysis to identify malignant cells within the specimen may not obviate the need for core or excisional biopsy of a suspicious mass. The chance of sampling error can be greatest in small tumors that elicit a fibrous response. These tumors often have a paucity of tumor cells. Most of the tumor mass-effect and surrounding tissues are formed of collagenous fibrous tissue.

H. Automated Spring-Loaded Core Biopsy

Percutaneous core biopsy techniques obtain several cores of tissue from an indeterminate or suspicious breast mass for histologic sampling. Accurate histologic diagnosis of a benign mass can obviate the need for an excisional biopsy. Core biopsy techniques can be performed with ultrasound or with mammographic stereotactic-guidance. When vacuum-assisted core biopsy systems are not available, breast core biopsies can be performed using an automated spring-loaded device.

Advantages of spring-loaded core biopsy compared to FNAB include:
*   Tissue cores provide more specimen and reduce sampling errors
*   Histologic sampling allows more reliable differentiation between in-situ and invasive cancers

Disadvantages of spring-loaded core biopsy compared to FNAB include:
*   More traumatic
*   Can require several insertions of needle
*   Longer wait for histologic results

General Procedure Description:
*   Requires local anesthetic; often small scalpel nick
*   Utilizes 14-18 gauge automated, spring-loaded needle biopsy gun or needle apparatus
*   Can require multiple insertions of the needle if introducer is not used
*   Needle is advanced in line with the mass (line-of-fire). Activation of the spring-loaded mechanism "fires" the biopsy needle into mass and quickly acquires a 10- 20mm long tissue core.
*   Needle placement parallel to the chest wall or skin reduces the risk of pneumothorax.
*   Approximately 3-5 cores are obtained, placed in formalin, and sent for histologic analysis
*   Hand-held pressure over the biopsy site reduces bleeding.

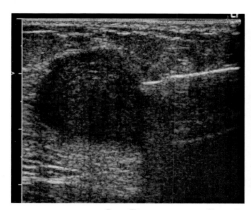 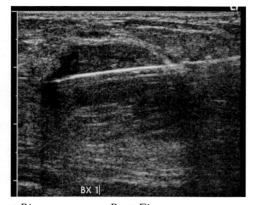

Pre-Fire   Core Breast Biopsy   Post-Fire
Automated Spring-loaded Device

Some false-negative diagnoses have been reported from tissue cores obtained of small breast cancers when using a spring-loaded automated core biopsy device. Large core biopsy such as vacuum-assisted biopsy, is often preferred for masses measuring < 1.5cm in diameter.

I. Vacuum-Assisted Core Biopsy

Vacuum-assisted breast (VAB) biopsy is a minimally invasive technique that retrieves relatively large tissue cores for histologic analysis. Several companies manufacture directional VAB devices for use with stereotactic, MRI, or ultrasound-guidance. US-guided VAB is often used to biopsy small indetermine or suspicious solid masses (< 1.5 cm in diameter) and certain complex lesions. Stereotactic guidance is preferred for biopsy of suspicious microcalcifications unless well seen on a sonogram.

Advantages of VAB compared to standard core biopsy include:
- Larger cohesive tissue cores reduce sampling errors (8, 9, 10, 11 guage depending on manufacturer)
- Single needle insertion
- Small lesion may be completely removed in some cases

Disadvantage VAB compared to standard core biopsy include:
- More expensive and often less available
- Possible higher chance of bleeding at biopsy site
- May be contraindicated for superficial mass or mass near implant

General Procedure Description (US-guided mammotomy):
- Requires local anesthesia, and a small scalpel skin nick
- A hand-held biopsy probe is attached to a vacuum console.
- An 11-gauge needle probe is typically used. (8g - 14g available)
- Using US-guidance, the needle probe is advanced directly under the mass. The probe aperture is opened and aligned under the lesion. (The opened aperture produces a "ring-down" artifact that helps to identify the probe aperture.)
- Vacuum suction pulls the specimen into the probe aperture.
- A rotating cutter severs the tissue and the vacuum pulls the specimen into a collection chamber without removal of the probe.
- Multiple consecutive samples are obtained in a clock-wise manner by rotating the aperture.
- A metallic clip can be deployed to mark the biopsy site for x-ray localization. (The clip is embedded in a rod-shaped collagen/gel pledget that is echogenic on ultrasound.)
- After the biopsy, pressure is applied over the site to reduce bleeding.

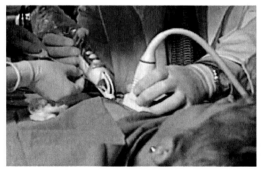

Mammotome vacuum-assisted biopsy done with free-handed technique.

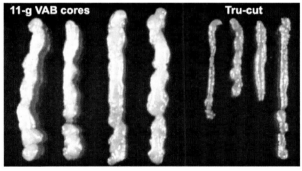

VAB provides larger and more cohesive tissue cores than from standard core biopsy techniques.

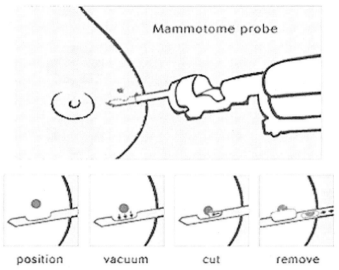

position   vacuum   cut   remove

www.breastbiopsy.com

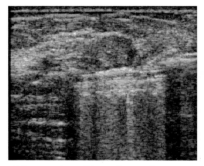

Mammotome® probe under mass Ring-down artifact denotes location of aperture.

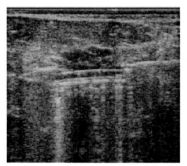

Vacuum suction pulls mass into aperture.

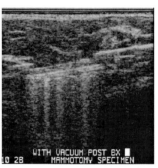

Mass no longer seen after multiple cores removed.

Images courtesy: Cindy Rapp, BS, RDMS

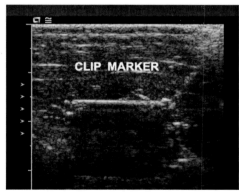

Ultrasound appearance of gel marker containing metallic clip.

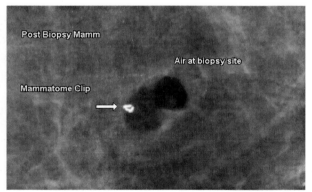

Mammogram appearance of metallic clip at VAB site with air at biopsy location.

J. Advanced Breast Biopsy Instrumentation (ABBI)

The ABBI device requires mammographic stereotactic guidance for insertion of a 0.5 cm - 2.0 cm cutting cannula to excise up to a 2.0 cm single core of breast tissue for diagnostic sampling.

Advantages of ABBI compared to other core biopsy techniques include:
- Large specimen reduces sampling error
- Diagnostic procedure with ability to fully excise small lesion

Disadvatages of ABBI include:
- Limited availability; can be expensive
- Requires radiologist and surgeon
- Removal of large specimen can increase bleeding, scarring
- Removes more normal tissue in path of mass than standard core bx.
- Requires stitches at biopsy site
- Surgical excision is still required for malignancy

General Procedure Description:
- Outpatient procedure; requires local anesthetic.
- Utilizes a prone stereotactic localization table together with an ABBI cannula device for core biopsy. Cutting cannula allows removal of either a 0.5 cm, 1.0 cm, 1.5 cm, or 2.0 cm tissue core.
- After stereotactic localization of the mass, a surgical incision is made in the breast. A rotating, cylindrical blade is inserted through the incision and advanced until the lesion is included in the core.
- An integrated diathermy wire severs the deep end of the full tissue core and the lesion is withdrawn.
- Mammography is performed to ensure complete removal of mass.
- Specimen radiography is performed of the excised tissue core.
- The specimen is then sent for histopathologic analysis.
- The incision site is sutured.

Although ABBI can completely excise a small lesion, it is considered a diagnostic, rather than an excisional, biopsy device by the FDA.

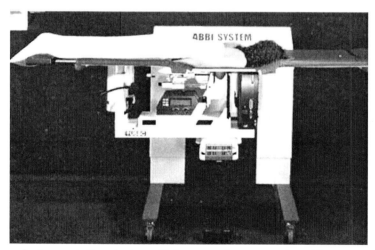

Advanced Breast Biopsy Instrumentation device with integrated stereotactic guidance system. (www.ussurg.com)

K. Pre-Operative US-Guided Localization

Pre-operative placement of a percutaneous needle wire and or methylene blue dye provides a visible guide for the surgeon to locate a nonpalpable breast mass for surgical excision. Stereotactic guidance is preferred for localizing microcalcifications.

The surgeon may prefer needle wire placement along the shortest path to the lesion. This is usually accomplished by advancing the localization needle in a near vertical approach towards the mass. However, this approach makes delineation of the needle shaft difficult during ultrasound guidance because of the steep angle of incidence. The surgeon removes the mass, along with wire or dye.

For superficial lesions, it is acceptable to "X" mark the skin overlying the lesion rather than placing a wire. The distance from the skin to the lesion should be noted for the surgeon.

The excised specimen can be radiographed or scanned in a saline bath with sonography to confirm the presence of the suspicious findings.

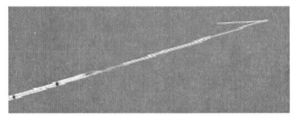

Kopan's localization wire.

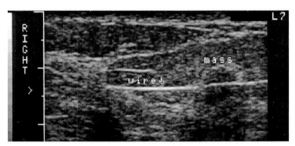

Localization wire in mass. Wire is easily seen since advanced parallel to the transducer.
However, the surgeon may prefer a shorter path for wire placement.

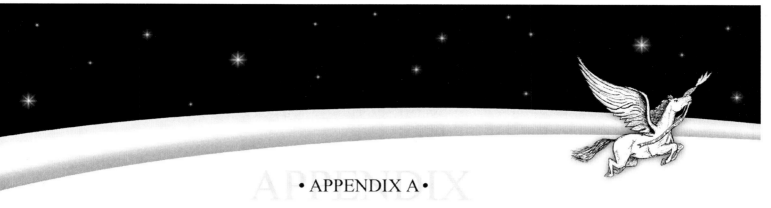

• APPENDIX A •

Review Test Questions

Instrumentation And Technique

1. A transducer suitable for high-resolution breast imaging is:
   a. 3.5 MHz, convex array
   b. 5.0 MHz, vector format
   c. 7.5 MHz, annular array
   d. 12.0 MHz, linear array
   e. 10.0 MHz; sector format

2. Use of a high frequency transducer to image the breast results in:
   a. Better sound penetration
   b. Poorer axial resolution
   c. Faster sound propagation
   d. Greater sound attenuation

3. A wide range of frequencies emitted by a high-frequency, pulsed- wave transducer is termed:
   a. Resonance frequencies
   b. Broad bandwidth
   c. Fremitus
   d. Harmonics

4. Identify the equipment control that directly affects the intensity of the sound beam emitted by the transducer.
   a. Overall gain
   b. Time gain compensation
   c. Dynamic range
   d. Output power

5. The use of multiple transmit zones results in:
   a. Improved sound penetration
   b. Slower frame rates
   c. Weaker sound intensity
   d. Higher frequency

6. Which of the following system controls does NOT affect echo brightness?
   a. Dynamic range
   b. Overall (receiver) gain
   c. Frame rate
   d. Time gain compensation
   e. Output power

7. Excessive use of overall receiver gain can cause:
   a. Failure to detect echoes within a solid mass
   b. Production of false echoes within a cyst
   c. Reduction in sound penetration
   d. Poor focusing
   e. Slice thickness artifacts

8. Time gain compensation is an equipment control that allows:
    a. Uniform amplification of all echoes received by the transducer
    b. Selective amplification of echoes to compensate for attenuation losses
    c. Alteration of sound beam intensity transmitted from the transducer
    d. Production of harmonic frequencies

9. The elevation plane of a conventional (1-D) linear array transducer refers to:
    a. Fixed focus in the short axis imaging plane
    b. Fixed focus in the lateral plane
    c. Variable focusing in the axial plane
    d. Electronic steering in the axial plane

10. Frame rate is affected by the following, EXCEPT:
    a. Number of focal zones
    b. Image depth
    c. Frequency
    d. Image size
    e. Line density

11. Which of the following Doppler method is LEAST angle dependent, thus allowing better demonstration of small, tortuous blood vessels?
    a. Spectral
    b. Color flow mode
    c. Power (energy) mode
    d. Continuous wave

12. The elevation focus of a conventional high-frequency linear transducer designed for breast imaging is fixed at a depth of approximately:
    a. 0.5 cm
    b. 1.5 cm
    c. 3.0 cm
    d. 4.0 cm

13. Indications for breast sonography include the following, EXCEPT:
    a. Initial evaluation of a palpable mass in female under age 30
    b. Characterization of a mammographic mass
    c. Screening for suspicious microcalcifications
    d. Needle guidance during aspiration or biopsy
    e. Evaluation of implant complications

14. A mass located at 9:00 (clock-face position) in the right breast is positioned:
    a. Superior to the nipple
    b. Inferior to the nipple
    c. Lateral to the nipple
    d. Medial to the nipple
    e. Subareolar

15. What patient position is best suited for ultrasound examination of an upper outer quadrant breast mass.
    a. Prone
    b. Ipsilateral posterior oblique
    c. Supine
    d. Contralateral posterior oblique

Pegasus Lectures, Inc.

16. Which artifact represents a decrease in echo amplitude beneath a strongly attenuating breast mass?
    a. Aliasing
    b. Reverberation
    c. Shadowing
    d. Enhancement

17. Identify the scan plane best suited for evaluation of the major lactiferous ducts.
    a. Longitudinal
    b. Transverse
    c. Antiradial
    d. Radial
    e. Coronal

18. The thickness of an acoustic standoff pad for breast sonography should not exceed:
    a. 0.5 mm
    b. 1.0 cm
    c. 1.0 mm
    d. 2.0 cm
    e. 3.0 mm

19. What structure should be demonstrated to ensure adequate sound penetration of the entire breast?
    a. Subcutaneous fat
    b. Superficial fascial layer
    c. Parenchyma
    d. Pectoralis muscle

20. The ability of an ultrasound system to distinguish anatomic structures based on variations in echo brightness is termed:
    a. Contrast resolution
    b. Spatial resolution
    c. Axial resolution
    d. Lateral resolution
    e. Elevational resolution

21. Which of the following would diminish blood flow detection in a breast mass when using color-flow Doppler?
    a. Applying excessive transducer pressure
    b. Using low flow velocity settings
    c. Optimizing the Doppler angle
    d. Reducing size of the Doppler box to the region on interest
    e. Increasing gain settings, without introducing artifacts

22. Doppler helps to differentiate:
    a. Blood vessels from ducts
    b. Hypervascularity from normal vascularity
    c. Papilloma from inspissated material in a duct
    d. Complicated cyst from a markedly hypoechoic solid mass
    e. All of the above

23. Using current standards of practice, the echogenicity of a breast mass is described in comparison to that of:
    a. Fat
    b. Fibroglandular tissue
    c. Muscle
    d. Skin

24. On a sonogram, the location of a breast lesion is annotated " L 1:30 1B RAD". All of the following correctly describe either the lesion's location or the scan plane, EXCEPT:
    a. Left breast
    b. Mid upper outer quadrant
    c. Inner third of breast
    d. Deep third of breast near the chest wall
    e. Radial scan plane

25. Which of the following is FALSE regarding the use of transducer compression during breast sonography?
    a. Decreases breast tissue thickness, thus allowing better sound penetration
    b. Decreases critical angle shadowing from Cooper's ligaments
    c. Assesses lesion compressibility
    d. Improves Doppler detection of blood flow

26. Identify the artifact indicated by the arrow on the sonogram.
    a. Reverberation
    b. Shadowing
    c. Enhancement
    d. Refraction
    e. Grating lobe

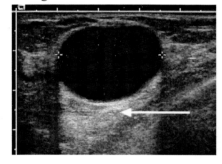

27. Identify the artifact seen along the anterior surface of the implant.

    a. Reverberation
    b. Shadowing
    c. Enhancement
    d. Refraction
    e. Grating lobe

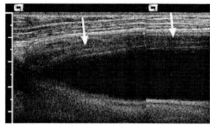

Anatomy

28. The function of the adult female breast is to produce:
    a. Estrogen
    b. Progesterone
    c. Milk
    d. Prolactin
    e. Oxytocin

29. During embryologic development of the breast, bilateral milk lines extend from the:
    a. Axilla to the inguinal region
    b. Axilla to the umbilicus
    c. Sternum to the umbilicus
    d. Sternum to the symphysis pubis

30. What structure contains the functional epithelial elements of the breast?
    a. Lobe
    b. Extralobular stroma
    c. Fat
    d. Dermis
    e. Montgomery gland

31. Identify the components of the terminal duct lobular unit.
    a. Excretory duct and lactiferous sinus
    b. Main duct and ampulla
    c. Acini and intralobular stroma
    d. Extralobular terminal duct and a lobule
    e. Segmental duct and excretory duct

32. Precocious puberty is more likely to be associated with:
    a. Premature development of both breasts
    b. Unilateral early ripening
    c. Amastia
    d. Congenital nipple inversion
    e. Athelia

33. The skin of the breast is composed of the:
    a. Pectoral and deep fascial layers
    b. Epidermis and Montgomery glands
    c. Epidermis and dermis
    d. Epithelium and myoepithelium

34. Normal skin thickness is typically equal to or less than:
    a. 0.5 mm
    b. 1.0 cm
    c. 2.0 mm
    d. 3.0 cm
    e. 4.0 mm

35. The mammary (parenchymal) layer of the breast contains the following structures, EXCEPT:
    a. Subcutaneous fat
    b. Lobes
    c. Lactiferous ducts
    d. Terminal duct lobular units
    e. Acini

36. Suspensory, dense connective tissue septa of the breast are called:
    a. Cooper's ligaments
    b. Terminal duct lobular units
    c. Intralobular stroma
    d. Montgomery glands
    e. Tail of Spence

37. Which of the following structures will display the greatest echogenicity?
    a. Duct epithelium
    b. Dense fibrous stromal tissue
    c. Fat
    d. Blood
    e. Loose intralobular stroma

38. A normal, intramammary lymph node typically displays the following sonographic features, EXCEPT:
    a. Oval, reniform shape
    b. Hypoechoic outer cortex
    c. Hypoechoic fatty hilum
    d. Doppler flow within the fatty hilum
    e. Well-circumscribed margins

39. Identify the breast structure indicated by the arrow on the sonogram.
    a. Skin
    b. Subcutaneous fat
    c. Fibroglandular tissue
    d. Retromammary fat
    e. Pectoralis muscle

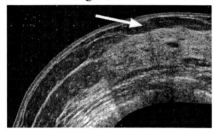

40. Identify the breast layer indicated by the arrow on the sonogram.
    a. Skin
    b. Subcutaneous fat
    c. Mammary
    d. Retromammary fat
    e. Pectoral

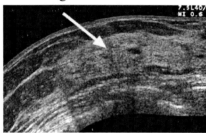

41. Identify the number of lobes in the female breast.
    a. 5 - 10
    b. 15 – 20
    c. 20 – 35
    d. 30 – 40

42. Primary sources of blood to the breast are the:
    a. Lateral thoracic and internal mammary arteries
    b. Axillary and brachial veins
    c. Thoracoacrominal and intercostals arteries
    d. Internal mammary and thoracoacromial veins

43. Identify the nodes that drain the majority of lymph from the breast.
    a. Supraclavicular
    b. Intercostal
    c. Axillary
    d. Internal mammary
    e. Rotter's

44. A breast duct focally widens beneath the areola at the:
    a. Lactiferous sinus
    b. Lobule
    c. Acini
    d. Montgomery gland

45. The presence of accessory nipples at a point along the milk line describes:
    a. Polymastia
    b. Polythelia
    c. Amazia
    d. Athelia

46. Extension of the glandular tissue into the axillary region is called:
    a. Axillary adenopathy
    b. Axillary tail of Spence
    c. Montgomery gland
    d. Papillomatosis

47. What cells line the inner portion of a breast duct?
    a. Epithelial
    b. Myoepithelial
    c. Cuboidal
    d. Squamous

48. Identify the tiny, milk producing structures in the lactational breast.
    a. Lactiferous ducts
    b. Acini
    c. Myoepithelial cells
    d. Sebaceous glands
    e. Montgomery glands

49. The mammary layer of the breast is enclosed between the:
    a. Skin and the subcutaneous fat
    b. Superficial and deep layers of the superficial fascia
    c. Premammary fascia and the superficial veins
    d. Retromammary fascia and the retromammary fat
    e. Intralobular stroma and the lobule

50. Two-thirds of the breast lies anterior to what muscle?
    a. Serratus anterior
    b. External oblique
    c. Pectoralis minor
    d. Pectoralis major
    e. Internal mammary

51. Normal breast structures that can simulate pathology include the following, EXCEPT:
    a. Costal cartilages
    b. Critical angle shadowing from Cooper's ligaments
    c. Isolated fat lobule surrounded by fibroglandular tissue
    d. Reverberation artifact

52. Branches of what nerve primarily innervate the breast?
    a. Brachial
    b. Intercostal (thoracic)
    c. Radial
    d. Pectineus
    e. Obturator externus

53. Identify the structure indicated by the arrows on the sonogram.
    a. Cooper's ligament
    b. Terminal duct lobular unit
    c. Intralobular stroma
    d. Lactiferous duct
    e. Artery

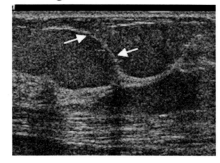

54. Identify the breast structures indicated by the arrows on the sonogram.
    a. Sebaceous glands
    b. Lactiferous ducts
    c. Microcysts
    d. Acini
    e. Interlobular stroma

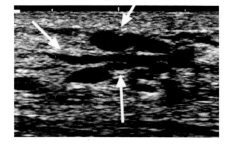

55. Identify the structure indicated by the arrow on the schematic.
    a. Lobule
    b. Main lactiferous duct
    c. Acini
    d. Excretory duct
    e. Extralobular duct

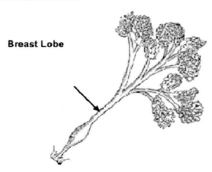

56. Identify the structure indicated by the arrow and bracket on the schematic.
    a. Lobule
    b. Main lactiferous duct
    c. Acini
    d. Excretory duct
    e. Dense interlobular stroma

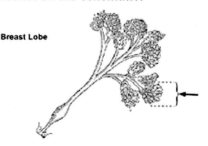

Sonographic-Mammographic Correlation

57. The following masses or tissues are "water density" on a mammogram, EXCEPT:
    a. Lipoma
    b. Fibroadenoma
    c. Carcinoma
    d. Cyst
    e. Fibroglandular tissue

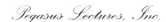

58.	The main purpose of screening mammography is to:
	a.	Evaluate breast secretions
	b.	Detect breast cancer in the asymptomatic patient
	c.	Differentiate cysts from solid masses
	d.	Biopsy an indeterminate mass
	e.	Evaluate silicone implants

59.	The standard views for screening mammography are:
	a.	Mediolateral oblique; True 90^0 lateral
	b.	Craniocaudad; Cone compression
	c.	Mediolateral oblique; Cone compression
	d.	Mediolateral oblique; Craniocaudad
	e.	Eklund view; Exaggerated craniocaudad

60.	On a mediolateral oblique mammogram, the side marker is placed by the:
	a.	Medial breast
	b.	Inferior breast
	c.	Axillary (upper outer) region of the breast
	d.	Nipple
	e.	Pectoralis muscle

61.	Correlation of the sonographic and mammographic features of a mass should include:
	a.	Size and shape
	b.	Margin characteristics
	c.	Location within breast
	d.	Density of the surrounding tissues
	e.	All of the above

62.	The earliest sign of cancer on a mammogram is:
	a.	Spiculated mass
	b.	Radiopaque asymmetric density
	c.	Cooper's ligament retraction
	d.	Microcalcifications
	e.	Skin thickening

Benign Vs. Malignant Descriptors -Features

63.	ACR BI-RADS® Category 3 classification indicates findings are:
	a.	Negative
	b.	Benign
	c.	Probably benign
	d.	Moderately suspicious of malignancy
	e.	Highly suggestive of malignancy

64.	Terms used to describe a mass that is oval in shape include the following, EXCEPT:
	a.	Ellipsoid
	b.	Elliptical
	c.	Egg-shaped
	d.	Irregular

65.	A well-defined mass that is sharply demarcated from surrounding tissues is described as being:
	a.	Circumscribed
	b.	Indistinct
	c.	Angular
	d.	Microlobulated
	e.	Spiculated

66. A breast mass that is more echogenic that normal breast fat is termed:
    a. Anechoic
    b. Hyperechoic
    c. Hypoechoic
    d. Markedly hypoechoic
    e. Isoechoic

67. Primary sonographic features of a breast mass include the following, EXCEPT:
    a. Shape
    b. Margin definition
    c. Echogenicity
    d. Attenuation effects
    e. Skin retraction

68. Benign sonographic features of simple breast cyst include the following, EXCEPT:
    a. Round or oval shape
    b. Thick, isoechoic walls
    c. Absent internal echoes
    d. Distal sound enhancement
    e. Thin, bilateral edge shadowing

69. Individual malignant sonographic features of a solid breast mass include the following, EXCEPT:
    a. Spiculation
    b. Angular margins
    c. Marked hyperechogenicity
    d. Acoustic shadowing
    e. Microcalcification

70. Uniform distribution and intensity of internal echoes describes:
    a. Heterogenicity
    b. Homogenicity
    c. Complex pattern
    d. Attenuation
    e. Enhancement

71. Which of the following is NOT a benign sonographic feature of a solid breast mass?
    a. Ellipsoid shape
    b. Wider-than-tall
    c. No more than three macrolobulations
    d. Complete, thin echogenic pseudocapsule
    e. Central acoustic shadowing

72. What sonographic finding correlates with a palpable lump that is caused by benign fibrous stomal tissue?
    a. Uniform, marked hyperechogenicity
    b. Ellipsoid
    c. Wider-than-tall
    d. Macrolobulation
    e. Thin echogenic pseudocapsule

73. A thin echogenic pseudocapsule around a benign solid breast mass represents:
    a. A noninfiltrative rim of compressed tissue
    b. An infiltrative zone extending into surrounding tissues
    c. Reactive fibrosis
    d. Inflammation of surrounding tissues
    e. Necrosis

74. A thick echogenic halo around a malignant mass likely represents:
   a. A noninfiltrative rim of compressed tissue
   b. The infiltrative border of the mass
   c. Tumor extension into a single duct
   d. Necrosis
   e. Hypovascularity

75. A mass that is "wider-than-tall" is likely to be:
   a. Round
   b. Angular
   c. Oriented parallel to the skin
   d. Isoechoic
   e. Indistinct

76. Architectural distortion is a term that describes:
   a. Disruption of normal anatomic planes
   b. Skin thickening
   c. Short surface undulations
   d. Indistinct margins of a mass
   e. Circumscribed margins

77. Microcalcifications display the following features, EXCEPT:
   a. Measure less than 0.5mm in size
   b. Cast acoustic shadows
   c. Suspicious finding for malignancy
   d. Better seen in hypoechoic mass than in nondistended duct

78. Sonographic features of breast infection and edema include the following, EXCEPT:
   a. Increased echogenicity of the subcutaneous fat
   b. Skin thinning
   c. Abscess formation
   d. Tissue hypervascularity
   e. Dilated lymphatic channels; interstitial fluid

79. A mass that measures greatest in its anteroposterior (AP) dimension is:
   a. Taller-than-wide
   b. Round
   c. Macrolobulated
   d. Horizontally oriented
   e. Complex

80. Tumor extension from a mass into a single duct leading towards the nipple describes:
   a. Angular margins
   b. Spiculation
   c. Architectural distortion
   d. Branch pattern
   e. Duct extension

81. Tumor extension from a mass into multiple small peripheral ducts describes:
   a. Angular margins
   b. Spiculation
   c. Retraction
   d. Branch pattern
   e. Duct extension

82. Another term that describes irregular, jagged contours of a suspicious lesion is:
    a. Angular margins
    b. Spiculation
    c. Architectural distortion
    d. Branch pattern
    e. Duct extension

83. The finding with the highest positive predictive value for invasive cancer on a mammogram and a sonogram is:
    a. Angular margins
    b. Spiculation
    c. Acoustic shadowing
    d. Branch pattern
    e. Duct extension

84. In the fatty breast, hyperechoic straight lines are seen radiating out from the surface of a suspicious solid mass. This finding represents:
    a. Spiculation
    b. Branch pattern
    c. Angular margins
    d. Duct extension
    e. Cooper's ligament thinning

85. A small, hypoechoic, taller-than-wide, solid mass with indistinct borders is:
    a. Typical of fibrocystic change
    b. Characteristic of fibroadenoma
    c. Indicative of inflammation
    d. Suspicious for malignancy
    e. A normal finding

86. What finding(s) are most worrisome for papilloma or cancer in a patient with nipple discharge?
    a. Bilateral discharge
    b. Non-spontaneous flow
    c. Milky discharge from multiple duct orifices
    d. Bloody discharge from a single duct orifice

87. Malignant causes of skin thickening include the following, EXCEPT:
    a. Lymphatic obstruction
    b. Direct tumor invasion
    c. Heart failure
    d. Inflammatory carcinoma
    e. Diffuse metastatic disease

88. The surface of this benign mass is:
    a. Microlobulated
    b. Angular
    c. Macrolobulated
    d. Indistinct
    e. Spiculated

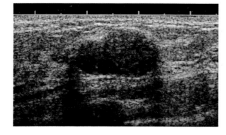

89. Identify the border characteristic (arrows) of this invasive breast cancer.
    a. Microlobulation
    b. Regular
    c. Thin echogenic capsule
    d. Thick echogenic halo
    e. Angular margins

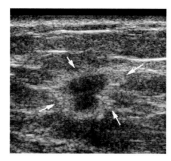

90. The attenuation effect associated with this breast cancer is:
    a. Normal transmission
    b. Sound enhancement
    c. Bilateral edge shadowing
    d. Mild, partial shadowing
    e. Pronounced shadowing

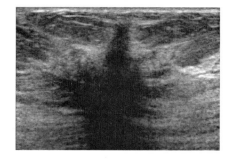

91. Skin changes demonstrated in this patient with inflammatory carcinoma include:
    a. Thinning and hyperechogenicity
    b. Thickening and hypoechogenicity
    c. Thickening and hyperechogenicity
    d. Thinning and isoechogenicity

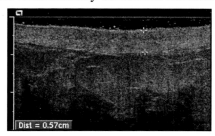

92. Features of this benign mass include the following, EXCEPT
    a. Wider-than-tall
    b. Ellipsoid
    c. Thick, echogenic halo
    d. Hypoechogenicity
    e. Normal sound transmission

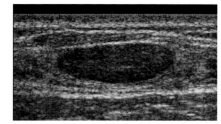

Benign Breast Pathology

93. What solid breast mass is most likely to be found in a woman less than 30 years of age?
    a. Phyllodes tumor
    b. Medullary carcinoma
    c. Invasive ductal carcinoma
    d. Juvenile papillomatosis
    e. Fibroadenoma

94. The lactational form of mastitis is called:
    a. Plasma cell
    b. Chronic mammary ectasia
    c. Puerperal
    d. Granulomatous
    e. Periductal

95. An associated complication of mastitis is:
    a. Hematoma
    b. Abscess
    c. Pneumothorax
    d. Seroma
    e. Radial scar

96. Identify the most common cause of bloody nipple discharge from a single breast duct.
    a. Fibrocystic change
    b. Intraductal papilloma
    c. Fat necrosis
    d. Fibroadenoma
    e. Invasive lobular carcinoma

97. Which mass commonly involves the dermal layer of the skin?
    a. Lobular neoplasia
    b. Hamartoma
    c. Fibroadenoma
    d. Sebaceous cyst
    e. Medullary carcinoma

98. A milk-filled retention cyst associated with lactation best describes a(n):
    a. Oil cyst
    b. Sebaceous cyst
    c. Epidermal inclusion cyst
    d. Hematocele
    e. Galactocele

99. The terminal duct lobular unit is the site of origin of the following breast pathologies or conditions, EXCEPT:
    a. Invasive ductal carcinoma
    b. Fibroadenoma
    c. Fibrocystic change
    d. Intraductal (large duct) papilloma
    e. Peripheral papillomatosis

100. Male breast enlargement due to proliferation of the subareolar ducts and surrounding stroma best describes:
    a. Pseudogynecomastia
    b. Gynecomastia
    c. Klinefelter's syndrome
    d. Montgomery glands
    e. Lobular neopasia

101. Which of the following is NOT a common clinical feature of fibroadenoma?
    a. Firm
    b. Fixed
    c. Movable
    d. Smoothly marginated

102. Features more worrisome for inflammation or infection of a cyst include the following, EXCEPT:
    a. Uniform, isoechoic wall thickening
    b. Fluid-debris levels
    c. Increased blood flow along cyst wall
    d. Thin, echogenic wall

103. What is most likely cause of this subareolar mass in a woman with nipple discharge?
    a. Fibroadenoma
    b. Medullary carcinoma
    c. Peripheral papillomatosis
    d. Mastitis
    e. Intraductal (large duct) papilloma

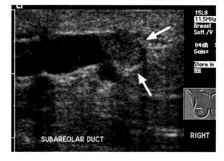

104. The mass shown on this sonogram in a 25 year old female is most likely to be a:
    a. Medullary carcinoma
    b. Fibroadenoma
    c. Hamartoma
    d. Phyllodes tumor
    e. Lipoma

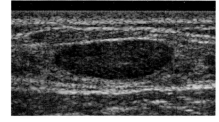

105. Benign breast masses with imaging features that can mimic carcinoma include the following. EXCEPT:
    a. Radial scar
    b. Fibrotic fat necrosis
    c. Granular cell tumor
    d. Diabetic fibrous mastopathy
    e. Lipoma

106. What feature of fibrocystic change is defined as an increase in the size and the number of the lobules?
    a. Adenosis
    b. Epithelial hyperplasia
    c. Duct dilatation
    d. Macrocysts
    e. Apocrine metaplasia

107. In what age group are breast cysts most common?
    a. 15-25
    b. 25-30
    c. 35-50
    d. 50-70

108. A collection of blood in the breast that results from trauma is:
    a. Abscess
    b. Lymphocele
    c. Hematoma
    d. Seroma
    e. Epidermal inclusion cyst

109. Artifactual echoes can be produced in breast cysts from:
    a. Excessive gain settings
    b. Reverberation
    c. Volume averaging
    d. Grating lobes
    e. All of the above

110. Features of a complex or a complicated cyst include the following, EXCEPT:
    a. Fluid-debris levels
    b Fat-fluid levels
    c. Low-level internal echoes
    d. Absent internal echoes
    e. Anechoic and echogenic components

111. Conditions related to breast trauma include the following, EXCEPT:
    a. Lipoma
    b. Fat necrosis
    c. Hematoma
    d. Scar
    e. Skin thickening

112. What traumatic breast condition can present as either a fibrotic, spiculated mass, or as an oil cyst?
    a. Galactocele
    b. Hematoma
    c. Fat necrosis
    d. Hamartoma
    e. Radial scar

113. Features of a post-operative scar include the following, EXCEPT:
    a. Shadowing that diminishes with transducer pressure
    b. Change in appearance in orthogonal scan planes
    c. Skin thickening; retraction
    d. Architectural distortion
    e. Hypervascularity

Malignant Pathology

114. The most common breast carcinoma is:
    a. Ductal carcinoma in situ
    b. Invasive lobular
    c. Invasive ductal
    d. Mucinous
    e. Medullary

115. Which breast cancer most often presents as an ill-defined or spiculated, hypoechoic, solid mass with distal acoustic shadowing?
    a. Medullary
    b. Mucinous
    c. Papillary
    d. Invasive ductal

116. Identify the most common extramammary primary cancer to metastasize to the female breast.
    a. Lung
    b. Melanoma
    c. Ovarian
    d. Gastric

117. An invasive cancer is more likely to be:
    a. Fixed and noncompressible
    b. Lobulated and rubbery
    c. Smooth and round
    d. Movable and compressible

118. Cancers that typically present as circumscribed tumors include the following, EXCEPT:
    a. Medullary
    b. Colloid
    c. Papillary
    d. Low-grade invasive ductal
    e. Phyllodes tumor

119. The presence of multiple cancer foci involving more than one breast quadrant is termed:
    a. Bilateral
    b. Multifocal
    c. Multicentric
    d. Proliferative

120. The most common location for male breast cancer is:
    a. Subareolar; eccentric to the nipple
    b. Upper outer quadrant
    c. Lower outer quadrant
    d. Upper inner quadrant
    e. Lower inner quadrant

121. The lifetime odds of an American woman developing breast cancer is:
    a. 1 in 20
    b. 1 in 15
    c. 1 in 8
    d. 1 in 5
    e. 1 in 3

122. Risk factors for breast cancer include the following, EXCEPT:
    a. Family history of breast cancer
    b. Personal history of atypical hyperplasia
    c. Early menopause
    d. Nulliparity
    e. Increasing age

123. A cancer that has spread past the duct wall and into the surrounding tissues is termed:
    a. In situ
    b. Intraductal
    c. Invasive
    d. Multicentric
    e. Multifocal

124. What invasive cancer is least likely to be detected on a mammogram or on clinical examination?
    a. Ductal
    b. Lobular
    c. Tubular
    d. Medullary
    e. Colloid

125. What noninvasive carcinoma is characterized by distension of ducts with necrotic, cheese-like material, and extensive calcifications?
    a. High nuclear grade (comedo) ductal carcinoma in situ
    b. Low nuclear grade ductal carcinoma in situ
    c. Lobular carcinoma in situ
    d. Cribiform

126. Which cancer is most likely to appear as a spiculated mass on imaging tests?
    a. Medullary
    b. Mucinous
    c. Intracystic papillary
    d. Invasive ductal
    e. Phyllodes

127. Which of the following is NOT a feature of medullary carcinoma?
    a. Rapid growth
    b. Circumscribed margins
    c. Hypoechoic; marked hypoechogenicity
    d. Central necrosis
    e. Acoustic shadowing

128. Another name for mucinous carcinoma is:
    a. Metaplastic
    b. Colloid
    c. Cystosarcoma
    d. Tubular
    e. Intraductal

129. A multifocal cancer refers to:
    a. Bilateral disease
    b. Tumor foci in multiple breast quadrants
    c. Multiple tumors within one breast quadrant
    d. Lymph node involvement
    e. Tumors separated by more than 5cm

130. Features of a phyllodes tumor include the following, EXCEPT:
    a. Circumscibed margins
    b. Potential to undergo malignant transformation
    c. Solid mass that can show internal cystic cavities
    d. Typically develops in teenage females
    e. Rapid growth rate

131. Characteristic features of inflammatory carcinoma include the following, EXCEPT:
    a. Orange peel appearance to skin
    b. Rapid, diffuse dissemination of breast cancer
    c. Tumor emboli within the lymphatics of the skin
    d. Lymphadenopathy
    e. Always low-grade invasive ductal carcinoma

132. Features of lymph node metastasis include:
    a. Enlargement
    b. Rounded shape
    c. Absent or displaced hilar fat
    d. Marked hypoechogenicity
    e. All of the above

Pegasus Lectures, Inc.

Other Imaging Modalities

133. What examination involves the retrograde injection of a radiopaque, contrast agent into a lactiferous duct?
    a. Scintimammography
    b. Galactography
    c. Venography
    d. Mammotomy

134. The first node to drain lymph from a primary breast cancer is called the:
    a. Sentinel node
    b. Parasternal node
    c. Axillary node
    d. Reactive node
    e. Terminal duct

135. What modality uses Gadolinium™ as a contrast agent to help detect breast cancer?
    a. Sonography
    b. Magnetic resonance imaging
    c. Computerized tomography
    d. Mammography
    e. Nuclear medicine

136. Characteristic features of an invasive breast cancer on contrast-enhanced MRI include:
    a. Rapid, moderate-to-marked tumor enhancement
    b. Slow, sustained tumor enhancement
    c. Absent rim enhancement
    d. Normal morphologic features
    e. All of the above

Implants

137. The ultrasound term that describes the appearance of an infolded implant shell surrounded by silicone in a patient with intracapsular rupture is:
    a. Echogenic noise
    b. Noose sign
    c. Stepladder sign
    d. Linguini sign
    e. Snowstorm sign

138. The most common type of silicone breast implant is:
    a. Single lumen; gel-filled
    b. Double lumen with outer saline chamber and inner silicone chamber
    c. Double lumen with outer silicone chamber and inner saline chamber
    d. Direct silicone injection
    e. None of the above

139. An implant used for postmastectomy reconstruction is typically placed:
    a. Beneath the pectoralis muscle
    b. In front of the retromammary fat
    c. Beneath the skin
    d. Inferior to the serratus muscle

140. What MRI term is used to describe intracapsular silicone implant rupture?
 a. Linguini sign
 b. Snowstorm sign
 c. Stepladder sign
 d. Silicone gel bleed
 e. All of the above

141. The feature shown on this sonogram in a patient with past history of extracapsular silicone implant rupture is:
 a. Echogenic noise sign
 b. Wavy-line sign
 c. Stepladder sign
 d. Linguini sign
 e. Noose sign

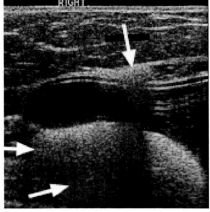

142. The findings on this sonogram in a patient with single lumen silicone implants is suggestive of:
 a. A normal exam
 b. Short radial fold
 c. Intracapsular rupture
 d. Herniation
 e. Fibrous encapsulation

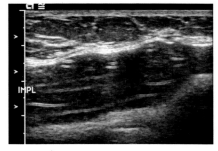

143. The rim of scar tissue that commonly forms around an implant is called:
 a. Capsular contracture
 b. Herniation
 c. Capsular rupture
 d. Fibrous capsule
 e. Siliconoma

Interventional Procedures

144. Identify the vacuum-assisted biopsy technique that extracts multiple 11-gauge tissue cores from a breast mass through a single needle insertion?
 a. Fine-needle aspiration
 b. Mammotome biopsy (Mammotomy)
 c. Advanced breast biopsy instrumentation
 d. Spring-loaded percutaneous core biopsy

145. To optimally visualize the needle tip and shaft during ultrasound-guided breast biopsy, the needle should be advanced:
    a. Parallel to the transducer face
    b. Perpendicular to the chest wall
    c. At a 20^0 angle
    d. At a 45^0 angle
    e. In any direction

146. A breast biopsy complication with associated symptoms of fever, elevated white blood count, and skin erythema is:
    a. Hematoma
    b. Abscess
    c. Lymphocele
    d. Seroma
    e. Galactocele

147. Which of the following biopsy complications is more likely to occur in a patient taking anticoagulants?
    a. Hematoma
    b. Infection
    c. Pneumothorax
    d. Allergic reaction
    e. Seroma

148. Which of the following masses would NOT need biopsy or aspiration?
    a. Suspicious enlarged lymph node
    b. Tender, enlarging cyst
    c. Complex cyst with cystic and solid components
    d. Suspicious solid lesion
    e. Asymptomatic, small, simple cyst

149. The least traumatic form of breast biopsy is:
    a. Advanced breast biopsy instrumentation
    b. Vacuum-assisted mammotomy
    c. Spring-loaded automated core biopsy
    d. Fine-needle aspiration biopsy

150. What percutaneous biopsy procedure has a greater chance of undersampling cancer cells within a mass?
    a. Fine-needle aspiration biopsy
    b. Automated spring-core biopsy
    c. Vacuum-assisted mammotomy
    d. Advanced Breast Biopsy Instrumentation

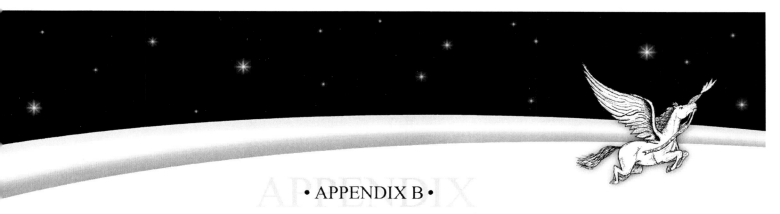

• APPENDIX B •

Review Test Questions Answer Key

1.	D	41.	B	81.	D	121.	C
2.	D	42.	A	82.	A	122.	C
3.	B	43.	C	83.	B	123.	C
4.	D	44.	A	84.	A	124.	B
5.	B	45.	B	85.	D	125.	A
6.	C	46.	B	86.	D	126.	D
7.	B	47.	A	87.	C	127.	E
8.	B	48.	B	88.	C	128.	B
9.	A	49.	B	89.	D	129.	C
10.	C	50.	D	90.	E	130.	D
11.	C	51.	D	91.	C	131.	E
12.	B	52.	B	92.	C	132.	E
13.	C	53.	A	93.	E	133.	B
14.	C	54.	B	94.	C	134.	A
15.	D	55.	B	95.	B	135.	B
16.	C	56.	A	96.	B	136.	A
17.	D	57.	A	97.	D	137.	C
18.	B	58.	B	98.	E	138.	A
19.	D	59.	D	99.	D	139.	A
20.	A	60.	C	100.	B	140.	A
21.	A	61.	E	101.	B	141.	A
22.	E	62.	D	102.	D	142.	C
23.	A	63.	C	103.	E	143.	D
24.	D	64.	D	104.	B	144.	B
25.	D	65.	A	105.	E	145.	A
26.	C	66.	B	106.	A	146.	B
27.	A	67.	E	107.	C	147.	A
28.	C	68.	B	108.	C	148.	E
29.	A	69.	C	109.	E	149.	D
30.	A	70.	B	110.	D	150.	A
31.	D	71.	E	111.	A		
32.	A	72.	A	112.	C		
33.	C	73.	A	113.	E		
34.	C	74.	B	114.	C		
35.	A	75.	C	115.	D		
36.	A	76.	A	116.	B		
37.	B	77.	B	117.	A		
38.	C	78.	B	118.	D		
39.	B	79.	A	119.	C		
40.	C	80.	E	120.	A		

Catherine Carr-Hoefer, RT, RDMS, RDCS, RVT

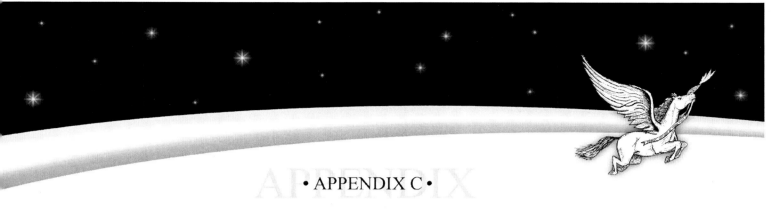

• APPENDIX C •

Glossary

Abscess

Localized collection of purulent material (pus) and a complication of breast infection (mastitis).

Absorption

Conversion of sound energy into heat as it travels through an acoustic medium. In soft tissue, absorption is the dominant factor causing sound beam attenuation. Absorption increases exponentially with increasing frequency.

Accuracy

Agreement of the test result with the true value of the sample. The accuracy of a test is determined by dividing the number of correct diagnoses by the total number of tests.

Acinus (acini)

Tiny, saccular, milk-producing gland(s) of the breast that are located in the breast lobule.

Acoustic impedance

Acoustic impedance (units of Rayls) equals the density of a medium times the propagation speed ($Z = p \, x \, c$). When there is a large difference between the acoustic impedances of two media at an acoustic interface, there will be a strong reflection.

Acoustic interface

Surface forming a boundary between media having different acoustic properties.

Adenocarcinoma

Malignant mass of epithelial origin that arises within the terminal duct lobular unit (within the ducts or lobule). Nearly all breast cancers are adenocarcinomas.

Adenoma

Benign mass composed of glandular (epithelial) tissue.

Adenosis

Overgrowth of the glands of the lobule. Characterized by an increase in the number and size of the acini and lobules, not in the number of cell layers. Adenosis is a feature of fibrocystic change.

Advanced Breast Biopsy Instrumentation (ABBI)

Specialized, stereotactic form of breast biopsy that uses a cutting cannula to remove up to a 2.0 cm single core of tissue for histologic analysis.

ALARA

A guideline to reduce patient exposure to ultrasound and stands for, "As Low As Reasonably Achievable."

Aliasing

An erroneous representation of the Doppler signal that occurs when the reflected frequency shift of a pulsed Doppler unit exceeds the Nyquist limit (i.e. PRF/2).

Amastia

Congenital absence of the breast tissue and nipple.

Amazia

Absence of the breast tissue.

Amplitude

The strength of the ultrasound beam. Amplitude is the maximum variation of an acoustic variable from its mean value. Increasing the amplitude of the echo signal will increase the echo brightness on the display.

Ampulla

(See lactiferous sinus)

Anechoic

Sonographic term that describes a structure that is echo-free. (This is a characteristic feature of a simple cyst.)

Angiogenesis (Neovascularity)

A biologic process causing the growth of new blood vessels to nourish cancer cells in response to chemical signals.

Angle of incidence

The angle at which an ultrasound beam strikes an acoustic interface. In Doppler, this is the angle at which the Doppler beam intersects the blood flow.

Angular margins

Refers to irregular, jagged contours of a mass. Angular margins increase the likelihood of malignancy of a solid mass.

Antiradial

The breast ultrasound scan plane that is orthogonal (90°) to the radial plane.

Artifact

Refers to any false information on the ultrasound image. An artifact does not correspond to a true anatomical structure at its location.

Athelia

Congenital absence of a breast nipple.

Attenuation

The reduction in wave amplitude and intensity as the sound beam travels through a medium. Factors leading to attenuation include sound absorption, reflection (specular; scattering) and refraction.

Axial resolution (depth, range, or longitudinal resolution)

The ability to image 2 closely spaced objects along the direction of the sound beam. Axial resolution is determined by the length of the ultrasound pulse and is equal to one-half the spatial pulse length (SPL/2). Axial resolution is a component of spatial resolution.

Pegasus Lectures, Inc.

Axillary dissection

A surgical procedure in which the lymph nodes in the armpit (axillary nodes) are removed and examined to determine the presence of nodal metastasis from a primary breast cancer. The cancerous lymph nodes are removed.

Backscatter

Sound energy that is reflected back towards the transducer from a scatterer.

Bandwidth

The range of frequencies emitted by a pulsed-wave transducer above and below the center (resonant) frequency. The bandwidth is the difference between the highest and lowest frequency found in a pulse. Broad bandwidth transducers emit a wide range of frequencies.

Benign

A non-malignant growth or condition that does not invade surrounding tissues or metastasize.

Bilateral

Refers to both sides of the body; or both breasts.

Biopsy

A procedure in which cells or tissue samples are removed from the body for microscopic examination to determine if cancer or other abnormal cells are present.

Branch pattern

Refers to tumor extension from surface of mass into smaller ducts leading away from the nipple (peripheral ducts). (As described by A.T. Stavros, MD)

BRCA 1; BRCA 2

Genes which, when damaged (mutated), place a woman at greater risk of developing breast cancer and/or ovarian cancer, than the general population.

Breast augmentation

Surgery to increase the size of the breast, typically involving placement of an implant.

Breast Imaging Reporting and Data System (BI-RADS®)

Reporting system developed by the American College of Radiology (ACR) to promote reporting consistency in the mammographic interpretation of breast disease. Assessment categories are based on the risk for malignancy.

Breast implant

A manufactured sac that is filled with silicone gel (a synthetic material) or saline (sterile saltwater). The sac is surgically inserted to increase breast size or to restore the contour of a breast following mastectomy.

Breast reconstruction

Surgery that rebuilds the breast contour after mastectomy using a breast implant or the woman's own tissue.

Carcinoma

A malignant tumor that arises from epithelial cells, such as those that line the ducts and lobules of the breast (adenocarcinoma). Nearly all breast malignancies are carcinomas.

Caudad
Refers to a direction toward the feet.

Center (resonance) frequency
The center frequency is the median frequency of the transmitted pulse.

Cephalad
Refers to a direction toward the head.

Colloid (mucinous) carcinoma
Special type of duct carcinoma composed of aggregates of tumor cells that float within mucin- filled compartments. Pure tumors are well-circumscribed and have a favorable prognosis.

Comedocarcinoma
Aggressive form of ductal carcinoma in situ. This intraductal tumor shows central necrosis associated with calcification.

Complex
Structure containing fluid and echogenic/solid components.

Contralateral
Refers to the opposite side (opposite breast).

Contrast imaging
Microbubble contrast agent is used to increase the amount of backscatter from the blood by increasing the acoustic impedance mismatch, thus allowing enhanced detection of tumor vascularity.

Contrast resolution
Refers to the ability of the ultrasound system to distinguish between structures based on variations in echo amplitude and brightness. (Measure of the sharpness of the lateral definition of the pulse.)

Measure of how well an ultrasound system can differentiate adjacent echoes of slightly different amplitudes, as well as large differences in echo amplitudes (such as a weak echo next to a strong one). Depends on the transducer type, frequency, and signal processing.

Cooper's ligaments
Dense, fibrous, connective tissue septa that are the supportive framework of the breast. These suspensory ligaments extend from the deep fascial layer to the skin. On a sonogram, Cooper's ligaments appear as thin hyperechoic bands, best seen when surrounded by fat.

Core biopsy
Use of a larger-gauge needle (than typically used for FNAB) to remove a cylindrical sample of tissue from a tumor for histologic analysis.

Critical angle / Critical angle shadowing
The angle of incidence at which there is total internal reflection. If the angle between the sound beam and a structure is far away enough from perpendicular, no sound energy or little sound energy travels distal to that interface, which results in a shadow. (Example: Cooper's ligament shadowing)

Cyst
Fluid-filled (serous) mass that typically result from obstruction of breast ducts within the terminal duct lobular unit.

186

Cystosarcoma phyllodes
(see phyllodes tumor)

Cytology
The study of cells, their origin, structure, function, and pathology.

Damping
Application of a material to the back of the transducer crystals to reduce ringing duration. Damping improves axial resolution by reducing pulse length.

Decibel (dB)
A unit for measurement of the relative intensity or amplitude of sound.

Desmoplasia (reactive fibrosis, fibroelastic host response)
A proliferation of fibrous tissue in and around a tumor that causes the tumor to become hard and fixed to surrounding structures. This fibrous reaction can thicken and shorten adjacent Cooper's ligaments, resulting in skin retraction. Desmoplastic tumors tend to feel larger on palpation than their size on a mammogram.

Doppler effect
A change in sound frequency (wavelength) that occurs whenever there is relative motion between the sound source and the reflector.

Double lumen implant
A type of breast prosthesis composed of two compartments (one saline; one silicone).

Duct ectasia
Distension of the breast ducts. Nonlactational causes include periductal mastitis, fibrocystic change, or secretory disease.

Duct extension
Tumor projection within a duct. Refers to tumor extension from the surface of a mass into a single duct leading toward the nipple. (A.T. Stavros, et al.)

Ductal carcinoma in situ (DCIS)
Malignant cells that proliferate within a duct without destruction of, or invasion past, the surrounding basement membrane. This noninvasive breast cancer is the earliest detectable form of breast cancer. Also termed intraductal carcinoma.

Ductography
A mammographic procedure to evaluate the lactiferous ducts using a water-soluble contrast agent.

Dynamic range
A parameter usually expressed in decibels that describes the ratio between the smallest to the largest signal strength level that the ultrasound system can handle without distortion. The displayed dynamic range is the range from the lowest grayscale level to the maximum grayscale brightness level on the image.

Echo palpation
Real-time scanning during palpation for direct correlation of clinical and sonographic findings. The palpable mass can be immobilized between two fingers while scanning over the mass.

Edema

Condition in which tissues contain excessive fluid resulting in swelling. Breast or skin edema can occur after trauma, infection, or from lymphatic obstruction.

Elastography

Modification of ultrasound exam that creates an image of a breast mass based on the relative stiffness of the tissue.

Elevation focus

Refers to the level of focus along the short axis of a linear array transducer; corresponds to the minimum slice thickness in the elevation plane. For a conventional high frequency, linear array breast transducer, the elevation focus is usually fixed at a depth of ~1.5cm by use of an acoustic lens.

Elevational resolution

Slice (section) thickness resolution.

Enhancement (acoustic)

An increase in echo amplitude from interfaces that lie beneath a non-attenuating or weakly attenuating structure (weak reflector or weak absorber).

Epithelial cells

Secretory cells comprising the inner layer of the breast ducts.

Epitheliosis

Epithelial hyperplasia that is characterized by an increase in the number of epithelial cell layers within the ducts and lobules. Can result in papillary formations (papillomatosis); feature of fibrocystic change.

Extracapsular implant rupture

Leakage of silicone into breast tissues from a breach in both the implant shell and the fibrous capsule.

Fascia

A sheet or thin band of fibrous tissue that covers muscles and various organs of the body. In the breast, the mammary layer is enclosed between the superficial and deep layers of the superficial fascia.

Fat necrosis

Nonsuppurative inflammatory process associated with destruction, liquefaction of fat cells, usually following trauma or infection. This benign condition can cause a fibrotic lesion with physical and imaging features that can mimic breast cancer, or present as an oil cyst.

Fibroadenolipoma (hamartoma)

A benign, intraglandular mass containing fibrous, glandular, and fatty breast tissue and surrounded by a pseudocapsule.

Fibroadenoma

A estrogen-induced,benign tumor composed of both connective (stromal) and ductal (epithelial) tissues. Represents the most common breast tumor in females under the age of 30 years.

Fibrocystic change / condition (FCC)

General term that describes a variety of benign alterations of the breast parenchyma related to hormonal changes. FCC is the most common, diffuse, benign breast disorder.

Pegasus Lectures, Inc.

Fibrous capsule (implant)
A shell of scar tissue that commonly forms around a breast implant as the body reacts to the foreign object. Fibrous encapsulation can lead to contracture.

Field of view (FOV)
The imaging plane demonstrated by a specific ultrasound transducer.

Fine needle aspiration biopsy (FNAB)
Multidirectional sampling of a mass using a small-gauge needle to withdraw cellular material for cytologic analysis.

Focus (focal zone)
The location where the sound beam reaches its minimum diameter and maximum intensity. Lateral resolution is best within the focal zone of the beam.

Frame rate
The number of frames displayed per second. Factors affecting frame rate of a real-time scanner include: depth of field, the total number of scan lines per image, and the number of focal zone. One frame constitutes one complete sweep of the ultrasound beam and will contain many pulse-listen cycles.

Fremitus
Color or power Doppler motion artifact produced from tissue vibration of the chest wall when the patient is asked to hum during breast scanning. This technique is used to better define the borders of masses and is helpful in differentiating normal from abnormal tissue.

Frequency
The number of cycles per unit time. The unit for frequency is the Hertz (Hz). One Hertz represents one cycle per second.

Gadolinium
Paramagnetic contrast agent used to enhance mass detection during magnetic resonance imaging (MRI).

Gain
Measure of the strength of the ultrasound signal. Can be expressed as the ratio of input to output in an amplifying system or in decibels. An increasing in receiver gain will increase the overall echo brightness.

Galactocele
A milk-filled retention cyst related to pregnancy and lactation. More likely to occur following abrupt cessation of lactation.

Galactography
(see ductography)

Gel Bleed
Presence of small amounts of silicone outside of an intact implant membrane due to the semipermeable nature of the elastomer shell.

Grating lobe
Off-axis beams of lower intensity sound energy generated by a multi-element transducer. A cause of spurious echoes on the ultrasound image.

Grayscale

Shades of gray displayed on the ultrasound image. For breast imaging, gain settings and grayscale levels should be adjusted so normal fat displays a medium-level gray shade.

Gynecomastia

Non-neoplastic male breast enlargement caused by proliferation of the subareolar ductal structures and the surrounding stroma.

Hamartoma

(see fibroadenolipoma)

Harmonic imaging

Mode of imaging in which the ultrasound system transmits at a given (fundamental) frequency and receives echoes at twice the transmit (second harmonic) frequency. This technique improves margin delineation during breast imaging and reduces artifacts.

Hematoma

A collection of blood outside a blood vessel due to vessel leakage or injury. Breast hematomas are typically related to direct trauma or surgery.

Hertz (Hz)

Unit of sound frequency that represents one cycle per second.

Heterogeneous

Refers to a medium composed of dissimilar elements resulting in a structure of non-uniform echo texture (containing hypo-,iso- and/or hyperechoic tissues).

Histology

The microscopic study of tissue.

Homogeneous

Refers to a medium of uniform texture and composition. Medium generating a uniform distribution and intensity of internal echoes.

Hyperechoic

Echogenicity of a structure that is of higher amplitude (brightness) than the surrounding tissue or a reference tissue.

Hyperplasia

An abnormal increase in the number of cells lining of the breast ducts or the lobules. By itself, hyperplasia is not cancerous, but when the proliferation (rapid growth) is marked and/or the cells are atypical (unlike normal cells), the risk of cancer developing is greater.

Hypoechoic

Echogenicity of a structure that is of lower amplitude than the surrounding tissue, or reference tissue.

Inflammatory carcinoma

Diffuse, aggressive carcinoma associated with tumor emboli within the dermal lymphatics that has a very poor prognosis.

Inframammary

Inferior to the breast.

190

Intensity

The total concentration of energy in an acoustic wave. (Intensity = Power (Watts) / Area) (Intensity ~ Amplitude^2)

Interlobular (extralobular) connective tissue

Dense fibrous tissue between the lobules.

Intracapsular implant rupture

Defect in the implant shell that allows silicone to leak between the implant shell and the intact, surrounding fibrous capsule.

Intralobular connective tissue

Loose connective tissue surrounding each breast lobule.

Invasive (infiltrating) carcinoma

Cancer that has spread beyond its area of origin to involve adjacent tissues. Such cancers gain access to the bloodstream and/or lymphatics and can metastasize.

Invasive ductal carcinoma

Refers to malignant epithelial cells that penetrate the basement membrane of the duct wall and invade the adjacent stroma. Such a cancer has the potential to metastasize. Invasive ductal carcinoma, not otherwise specified (IDC, NOS), is the most common breast malignancy and arises within the terminal ductal lobular unit.

Invasive lobular carcinoma

Cancer that arises within epithelium of the breast lobule and infiltrates the adjacent tissue. It is often difficult to detect by physical or mammographic examination. Represents the second most common invasive breast cancer. Tumor cells can infiltrate in single file rows (Indian files).

Ipsilateral

Term used to describe a structure on the same side.

Isoechoic

Echogenicity of a structure that is equal in amplitude to that of the surrounding tissues or of a reference tissue.

Kilohertz; KHz

Correlates to a sound frequency of one thousand cycles per second. (1 kHz = 1000 Hz)

Lactiferous sinus; ampulla

Focal dilatation of a lactiferous duct just beneath the areola here milk or secretions can accumulate.

Lateral

Anatomical term that describes a position away from the midline.

Lateral Resolution

The minimum separation necessary to distinguish two objects lying side by side in a direction perpendicular to direction of the sound beam. Lateral resolution is determined by the beamwidth.

Linear array transducer

Transducer with multiple rectangular elements arranged in a linear format; creates a rectangular image field.

Linguini sign

MRI term used to describe a collapsed breast implant shell suspended in silicone. This is a feature of intracapsular rupture.

Lipoma

A benign breast mass composed of fatty tissue.

Lobe

One of 15-20 segments of the breast that is radially arranges about the nipple. A lobe contains a ductal system that includes a main lactiferous duct, segmental ducts and smaller branches, as well as the terminal duct lobular units.

Lobular carcinoma in situ (LCIS)

Early type of noninvasive breast cancer that arises within the lobular epithelium. The preferred term for this condition is lobular neoplasia. LCIS places a woman at increased, future risk of developing an invasive breast cancer in either breast.

Lobule

Functional unit of the breast containing an intralobular terminal duct, ductules and associated acini. These lobular structures are surrounded by intralobular stroma.

Longitudinal

Anatomical term describing a position parallel to the long axis of the body.

Longitudinal wave

Wave in which the particle in the medium oscillates (back and forth) in the same direction as the wave propagation. Sound is a longitudinal, mechanical wave.

Lymphoma

A cancer arising from lymphocytes (a type of white blood cell) that usually develops in lymph nodes. The two main types are Hodgkin's disease and non-Hodgkin's lymphomas.

Lymphoscintigraphy

Nuclear medicine procedure that involves injection of a radiocolloid isotope to map lymph drainage from a primary breast cancer. This procedure allows the preoperative identification of the first lymph node (sentinel node) in the draining basin. Vital blue dye is an additional mapping agent.

Macrocalcifications

Coarse calcium deposits in the breasts (typically > 0.5mm); larger than microcalcifications. Macrocalcifications are associated with benign (non-cancerous) conditions and do not typically require a breast biopsy. Found in approximately 50% of women over the age of 50.

Macrolobulation

Refers to the gently-curving, smoothly lobulated contour of a breast mass.

Magnetic resonance imaging (MRI)

Non-ionizing technique that created cross-sectional images of the body by using a powerful magnet. Images are produced by computer analysis of radio frequency waves transmitted by the body. Breast coils are needed for breast imaging.

Malignancy

Term used to describe a mass of cancer cells. Malignant tumors may invade surrounding tissues or spread (metastasize) to distant areas of the body.

Mammary layer

The middle layer of the breast located between the subcutaneous and retromammary fat layers. This parenchymal layer of the breast contains glandular and stromal tissues.

Mammography

X-ray examination of the breast using specialized equipment. The breast tissue is compressed between the x-ray and compression plates to obtain a clear image of the interior structures of the breast. Screening mammography is used for early detection of breast cancer in women without any breast symptoms. Diagnostic mammography is used to characterize breast masses or determine the cause of other breast symptoms. (FFMD = Full-field Digital Mammography.)

Mammoplasty

Surgical procedure for breast augmentation or reduction.

Mammotomy

Breast biopsy procedure involving the insertion of 11-gauge needle probe (8-14g) to extract tissue cores or calcifications using vacuum suction assistance.

Mastectomy (radical; partial)

Surgical removal of all or part of the breast, and sometimes, adjacent tissue.

Mastitis

Inflammation or infection of the breast.

Matrix array transducer

Newer generation transducer with multiple rows of elements in grid pattern allowing focusing in elevation and lateral planes.

Mechanical wave

Wave that needs a medium in which to propagate (cannot propagate in a vacuum). Sound is a mechanical wave.

Medial

Anatomic term describing a position toward the midline.

Medullary carcinoma

An uncommon, special type of ductal carcinoma with lymphoid stroma that usually has well-circumscribed margins. This tumor tends to occur in women under the age 50 years and has a favorable prognosis.

Megahertz (MHz)

Correlates to a sound frequency of one million cycles per second. (1,000,000 Hz = 1MHz)

Metastasis

Spread of cancer cells to distant areas of the body by way of the bloodstream or lymphatics.

Microcalcifications
Tiny deposits of calcium measuring < 0.5mm. Malignant calcifications are typically intraductal and have varying presentations that include: a "cluster of pleomorphic calcifications (> 5 calcifications/cm^3 of tissue); dot-dash branching pattern and irregular shapes.

Microlobulation
Multiple small lobulations (undulations) along the surface of a mass.

Milk lines
Bilateral ectodermal ridges that extend from the axilla to the inguinal regions that are the embryologic sites of breast development.

Montgomery's glands
Sebaceous glands of the areola.

Multicentric breast cancer
Breast cancer occurring in multiple areas of a breast; in more than one breast quadrant. Tumors are generally separated by a distance ≥ 5cm. (Some references cite > 3cm separating distance.)

Multifocal breast cancer
Additional sites of breast cancer in the same quadrant as the primary tumor. Tumors are within 5cm of the primary tumor.

Myoepithelial cells
Outer cell layer of the breast ducts next to the basement membrane. These cells contain myofilaments that contract to transport milk from the acini through the ducts.

Needle aspiration
Percutaneous removal of fluid from a cyst or fluid-containing mass through a needle by application of suction from a syringe, vacutainer, or aspiration pump. If the needle is thin (small-gauge), the procedure is called a fine needle aspiration or FNA. The aspirate can be sent for cytologic analysis.

Neoplasm
An abnormal growth (tumor) that starts from a single altered cell, a neoplasm may be benign or malignant.

Noise
An ultrasound term referring to random, and usually undesirable signals.

Orthogonal scan planes
Ultrasound scan planes that are perpendicular (900; at right angles) to each other. (Examples: longitudinal and transverse; radial and antiradial)

Output power
Equipment control that affects the excitation voltage that drives the transducer crystals. A higher voltage will produce a stronger sound beam and increase the acoustic exposure to patient.

Overall gain
Receiver gain control that uniformly amplifies the amplitude of all received echo signals regardless of depth.

Pegasus Lectures, Inc.

Paget's disease of the nipple
Rare form of breast cancer that arises in the subareolar ducts and spreads to the skin of the nipple and areola. The affected skin has an eczema-like appearance and may appear scaly, reddened, or eroded.

Papillary carcinoma
Rare, special type of ductal carcinoma. Tumors can be in situ or invasive; solid or intracystic. Masses tend to occur in postmenopausal women and usually have a good prognosis.

Papilloma (intraductal; large duct papilloma)
Benign, proliferative epithelial tumor with a fibrovascular core that grows within a major lactiferous duct. This tumor is the most common cause of bloody nipple discharge.

Peau d'orange
French term that means "skin of the orange." This term describes the appearance of thickened, edematous skin of the breast with inversion of the pores. This finding is associated with lymphedema from such conditions as inflammatory carcinoma and mastitis.

Pectoralis major muscle
The main muscle lying posterior to the breast that runs obliquely from the mid-sternum to the humerus.

Periareolar
Around the perimeter of the areola.

Phyllodes tumor
Malignant counterpart of fibroadenoma, in which the stromal component can undergo malignant transformation and potentially metastasize. Previously known as cystosarcoma phyllodes.

Pneumocystography
A procedure in which air is injected into a breast cyst cavity following aspiration. The air allows mammographic evaluation of the cyst wall. Air injection can be therapeutic and reduce refilling of the cyst.

Polymastia
Accessory (supernumery) breasts.

Polythelia
Accessory (supernumery) nipples. Congenital condition occurring along the milklines.

Power Mode
Utilizes the color maps to display the amplitude of color Doppler signals (regardless of velocity).

Propagation Speed (Velocity)
The rate at which a sound wave travels through a medium. The propagation speed is affected by the stiffness (compressibility) and density of a medium. {Propagation speed (c) = frequency (f) x wavelength (λ)} The speed of sound though soft tissue is ~1540 m/s whereas silicone is ~ 1000 m/s.

Propagation Speed Error – artifact
Artifacts that results in a misregistration of a structure because the actual propagation velocity is not the assumed propagation velocity of 1540 m/s.

Pseudomass
False mass; structure or condition that mimics the presence of a breast mass.

Puerperal Mastitis
Breast inflammation that occurs during pregnancy and lactation. Represents the most common type of "acute" mastitis.

Pulsed Wave Doppler
A Doppler instrument which utilizes one transducer crystal to transmit and receive ultrasound pulses. Sampling the returning signal at a specific time interval allows flow to be assessed at determined sites and depths.

Radial
Breast ultrasound scan plane that is orthogonal (90^0) to the antiradial plane. The radial plane is oriented in the breast from the nipple towards the periphery like the "hands of a clock".

Radial Scar
Nontraumatic, benign elastoic lesion with spicules of proliferating epithelium that radiate out from a central fibrous core. Imaging features can mimic cancer.

Reflection
An event in which the sound wave changes direction so that some of the wave energy does not continue to propagate forward. Types of reflection include specular and scattering (back scatter; Rayleigh scatter). The amount of sound energy reflected is determined by the acoustic impedance mismatch, the incident angle, and the type of reflection.

Refraction
A change in direction (bending) of the sound beam as it crosses an interface. Refraction occurs when there is a change in propagation speed between the two media and when there is oblique incidence.

Refractive Edge Shadowing
Bending of sound beam and loss of sound energy causing a shadow. Encountered at curved edges of breast cysts and some solid masses, and with oblique incidence to Cooper's ligaments.

Retromammary fat layer (Retromammary Zone)
The deepest of the three main breast layers separating the mammary layer from the pectoralis major muscle. This layer is often thin and composed of adipose tissue and connective fascia.

Reverberation
Ultrasound artifact that represents multiple, repetitive reflections between two strong, specular reflectors. The "bouncing back and forth" between the transducer and the reflector increases travel time, causing the reverberating echoes to be displayed as parallel echoes at different depths on the image.

Sagittal
A longitudinal scan plane parallel to the median (midline) plane of the body. The median plane separates the body into right and left portions.

Sarcoma
A malignant tumor growing from connective tissues. Several types of sarcoma (such as angiosarcoma, liposarcoma, and malignant phylloides tumor) can develop in the breast. They are rare and differ in their prognosis.

Pegasus Lectures, Inc.

Scattering

A condition that occurs when the ultrasound beam strikes a reflector whose surfaces is rough relative to the wavelength. Rayleigh scattering occurs when the reflector is small in comparison to the wavelength (e.g., red blood cells). The sound beam is diffusely reflected and refracted in all directions as opposed to specular reflection in which sound is reflected in one direction.

Screening

The search for disease, such as cancer, in people without symptoms. Screening may refer to coordinated programs in large populations. The principal screening measure for breast cancer is mammography.

Sebaceous / epidermal cyst

Superfically located retention cyst that results from obstruction of a sebaceous gland or hair follicle.

Sentinel node

The first lymph node in the drainage basin of a primary breast cancer.

Sensitivity

The extent to which a diagnostic test correctly detects disease. Sensitivity indicates the frequency of positive test results in patients who have the specific disease being tested. A test's sensitivity is calculated by dividing the number of true positive tests by the number of all positive diagnoses (including true positive tests as well as false positive tests).

Seroma

A collection of serous fluid often seen trapped in a surgical site; usually forming after breast surgery or axillary dissection.

Shadowing (acoustic)

A reduction in echo amplitude or an absence of echoes from interfaces that lie behind a strong reflector or sound absorber.

Side Lobe

Lower intensity sound beams directed in regions other than the main beam axis that produce artifacts on the ultrasound image. Grating lobes are extra beams emitted from a multi-element transducer array.

Slice Thickness

The width of the ultrasound beam in the dimension perpendicular to the scanning plane (along the short axis of a linear array transducer).

Snowstorm sign

Unique ultrasound appearance of silicone within breast tissue or lymph nodes. Affected tissues appear echogenic and show "dirty shadowing" which obscures posterior structures.

Spatial compound imaging

Newer real-time technique that provides a single compound image created from multiple scan planes transmitted sequentially from different angles. Compound imaging improves the definition of the margins of masses, subareolar structures, and reduces artifacts.

Spatial resolution

Detail resolution for an ultrasound system that is measured in the axial and lateral (and elevational) planes.

Spatial Pulse Length
The length of an ultrasound pulse and is equal to the product of the wavelength and the number of cycles in a pulse.

Specificity
The ability of a diagnostic test to exclude the presence of disease and to detect normality. The specificity of a test is determined by dividing the number of true negative tests by the total number of negative diagnoses (this includes true negative tests as well as false positive tests).

Specular Reflector
Bright reflection from a smooth interface that is larger than the wavelength of the transmitted sound beam. With specular reflection, the sound strikes the target at perpendicular incidence and the sound is reflected back towards the transducer.

Spiculation
Fibrous bands (spicules) radiating out in straight lines from a central mass. A feature of invasive breast cancer. Ultrasound spiculation refers to alternating hypoechoic and hyperechoic bands radiating out perpendicularly from the surface of a mass (A.T. Stavros, et al.).

Stage
A term used to describe the extent of cancer. Staging of breast cancer is based on the size of the tumor, whether regional axillary lymph nodes are involved, and whether distant spread (metastasis) has occurred. Knowing the stage at diagnosis is essential in selecting the best treatment and predicting a patient's outlook for survival.

Standoff (acoustic)
Placement of a sound transmitting pad, or extra scanning gel to offset the transducer from the skin. Use of an acoustic standoff improves imaging the superficial breast structures by improving near field focusing and by reducing slice thickness artifacts.

Stepladder sign
Sonographic feature of intracapsular implant rupture seen as multiple, parallel, echogenic linear bands. These bands represent the infolded implant shell suspended within the silicone gel contained by the fibrous capsule. Also referred to as the parallel-line sign.

Stromal fibrosis
Represents an overgrowth of the fibrous connective tissues. This condition is a feature of fibrocystic change.

Subcutaneous fat layer
The most superficial of the three main levels of breast; located between the skin and mammary layer.

Suspicious
A breast abnormality that may indicate breast cancer. On a mammogram, these abnormalities may be lesions such as spiculated masses or clustered / pleomorphic microcalcifications.

Tail of Spence
Tongue-like extension of glandular tissue projecting towards or into the axilla.

Pegasus Lectures, Inc.

Taller-than-wide
Describes a breast mass that measures greater in its anteroposterior (AP) dimension than in either horizontal dimension. Such a mass is oriented with its longest axis perpendicular to the skin and is a feature suspicious for cancer.

Terminal duct lobular unit (TDLU)
The functional unit of the breast composed of the extralobular terminal duct and a lobule. The TDLU is the site of origin of most breast pathologies.

Time gain compensation (TGC); Depth gain compensation (DGC)
Receiver gain control that compensates for attenuation of the transmitted beam as sound travels through tissues. Operator can manually adjust the degree of amplification for a specific depth.

Transducer
A device that converts one form of energy into another form of energy.

Transducer (Ultrasound)
Piezoelectric crystal (s) produce a mechanical sound wave when excited by an electrical voltage and conversely produces an electrical voltage when acted upon by a mechanical sound wave.

Transverse rectus abdominus muscle (TRAM) flap procedure
Method of breast reconstruction in which tissue from the lower abdominal wall which receives its blood supply from the rectus abdominus muscle is used.

Ultrasound
Sound frequency above 20,000 Hertz (20 kHz); above the audible range. (Diagnostic medical ultrasound 2-17 MHz.)

Wavelength (λ)
The physical distance between cyclical wave peaks (one complete ultrasound compression and rarefaction cycle) within a medium. (Wavelength = propagation speed divided by frequency.) ($\lambda = c / f$) As frequency increases, wavelength decreases.

Wire (needle) localization
A procedure used to guide a surgical breast biopsy / lumpectomy of a nonpalpable mass, or suspicious area on imaging tests using a wire. A blue dye may added along the wire tract or used in place of a wire.

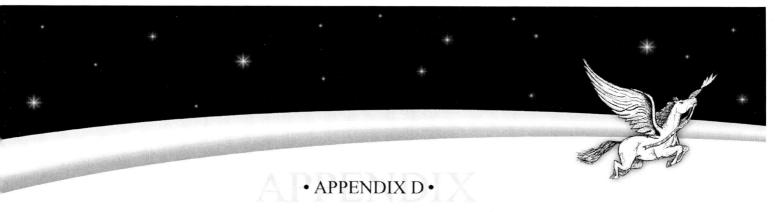

• APPENDIX D •

Major References

Berg WA, Birdwell RL et al. Diagnostic Imaging: Breast. Salt Lake City: Amirys; 2006

Cardenosa G. Breast Imaging Companion, 2nd ed. Philadelphia, Lippincott Williams & Wilkins; 2001.

Carr-Hoefer C. Breast Sonography. In: Kawamura D, ed. Abdomen and Superficial Structures. 2nd ed. Philadelphia: Lippincott; 1997.

Carr-Hoefer C. Breast Ultrasound Exam Simulation CD, SDMS / Pegasus Lectures, Inc., 2003.

Carr-Hoefer C, Grube JA. National Certification Examination Review: Breast ultrasound. Dallas, SDMS Publication, 2002.

Caskey CI, Berg WA et al. Imaging spectrum of extracapsular silicone: correlation of US, MR imaging, mammographic, and histopathologic findings. Radiographics 1999;19:s39-s51.

Dahnert W. Radiology Review Manual. 3rd ed. Baltimore: Williams & Wilkins; 1996.

Donegan WL, Spratt JS. Cancer of the Breast. Philadelphia: WB Saunders; 1995.

Glenn ME. The Breast. In: Hagen-Ansert SL, ed. Textbook of Diagnostic Ultrasonography. 5th ed. St.Louis: Mosby; 2001.

Hagen-Ansert SL, ed. Textbook of Diagnostic Ultrasonography. 5th ed. St.Louis: Mosby; 2001.

Heywang-Kobrunner SH, Dershaw DD, Schreer I. Diagnostic Breast Imaging. New York: Thieme; 2001.

Integrated Ultrasound Reference Guide, Vol 1, SDMS Educational Foundation

Lanfranchi ME. Breast Ultrasound. 2nd ed. New York: Thieme; 2000.

Madjar H, Jellins J. The Practice of Breast Ultrasound: Techniques, Findings, Differential Diagnosis. Stuttgart; New York: Thieme Publishers; 2000.

Mendelson EB, Berg WA, Merritt CR. Towards a standardized breast ultrasound lexicon, BI-RADS: ultrasound. Semin Roentgenol 2001;36(3)217-225.

Mendelson EB. The Breast. In: Rumack CM, Wilson SR, Charboneau JW, eds. Diagnostic Ultrasound. 2nd ed. St. Louis: Mosby; 1999.

Middleton MS, McMamara MP: Breast Implant Imaging. Philadelphia: Lippincott Williams & Wilkins; 2002.

Miele F., Ultrasound Physics and Instrumentation, 4th Edition: Pegasus Lectures; 2006

Rapp C. Sonography of the Breast. SDMS 17th Annual Conference Official Proceedings. Dallas, TX; 2000; 57-67.

Saslow D et al. American Cancer Society for Breast Cancer Screening with MRI as an adjunct to mammography; CA: Cancer JOurnal for Clinicians 2007; 57 (2): 75-89.

Stavros AT. Breast Ultrasound. Philadelphia, Lippencott Williams & Wilkins, 2004.

Stavros AT. Breast Ultrasound for Sonographers. SDMS 18th Annual Conference Official Proceedings. Dallas, TX; 2001; 33-45.

Stavros AT, Rapp C. US: Breast Ultrasound 2001. Audiovideo lecture presentation. TiP-TV™, GE Medical Systems, 2001.

Stavros AT, Thickman D, Rapp C, et al. Solid breast nodules: use of sonography to distinguish between benign and malignant lesions. Radiology 1995;196:123-134.

Tohno E, Cosgrove DO, Sloan JP. Ultrasound Diagnosis of Breast Disease. Edinburgh: Churchill Livingstone; 1994.

Vitale J. Breast Registry Review Syllabus.

Internet Resources

AIUM: The Standard for Performance of Breast Ultrasound Examination. December 2003 http://www.aium.org

American College of Radiology: ACR Practice Guidelines for the Performance of Breast Ultrasound Examination. Rev. 2007 http://www.acr.org.

Histology: http://mammary.nih.gov.com)

Imaginis: www.imaginis.com

Medcyclopaedia: www.amershamhealth.com

Philips Ultrasound: www.theonlinelearningcenter.com

The American Cancer Society: www.breastcare.com